CONSIDERING CANNABIS

The Mass Suffering of Humanity Depends on It!

David "PlayTime" Putvin

Published by
Hybrid Global Publishing
333 E 14th Street
#3C
New York, NY 10003

Manufactured in the United States of America, or in the United Kingdom when distributed elsewhere.

Putvin, David.
Considering Cannabis
    ISBN: 978-1-957013-61-9
    eBook: 978-1-957013-62-6
    LCCN: 2022920236

Cover design by: Jonathan Pleska
Copyediting by: Claudia Volkman
Interior design by: Suba Murugan

Disclaimer: *Considering Cannabis* does not provide dosage recommendations for any specific medical conditions. This book is designed to provide logical consideration and does not provide specific dosage recommendations for anybody.

Table of Contents

Introduction

Growing up in Utah, I thought Cannabis would be illegal forever. As a kid, I was told by religious leaders, family members, and other church members that Cannabis was poison to the body and would ruin my life. In my teens, I thought Cannabis was only good for managing pain if someone was nearing death and that recreational use was no different than abusing pain pills. Eventually, I realized that Cannabis is more like water. Just like water, Cannabis is beneficial to everyone—whether they like to drink water or not.

I was an MMA cage fighter from 2010–2019. I am happy I was able to retire by choice, and now I plan to continue doing Jiu-Jitsu until my body quits for good. I wanted to fight for the UFC, and I wanted to become famous for a specific reason: I wanted to be one of the best Jiu-Jitsu fighters ever so I could become a legendary spokesman for Cannabis and other psychoactive therapies. I was extremely dedicated to this goal, and I spent a lot of my life training and writing in preparation. I even went so far as to write my very own "Letter to Humanity," which I planned to announce after winning my first fight in the UFC. I wanted to publicly insist that every religious leader respect their followers by promoting the benefits of Cannabis. You see, I believe that Cannabis is not sinful, Cannabis has never been sinful, and Cannabis will never be sinful. Cannabis prohibition leads to the elimination of free will for every human who is wrongfully affected by laws based on greed and corruption. My "Letter to Humanity" is along those lines.

I dream of having private conversations with the pope, Dalai Lama, prophets, or any other religious leader who would be willing to meet with me. My intentions are to help end mass suffering in religious populations. I believe that my intentions are honest and could actually make a difference in the hearts and minds of religious leaders. These leaders are largely currently responsible for maintaining mass amounts of suffering for billions of people in this world due to the erroneous prohibition of Cannabis. I'd love the opportunity to meet any religious leaders who might be interested in sitting down face-to-face with me to discuss how together we can reduce mass suffering on Earth.

My intention is to make the message of Cannabis clear to everyone. Religious leaders need to be held publicly accountable for their disregard of the health of their religious members. Everyone should be protected in their pursuit of any religion they choose, and I don't think any religion or country should be allowed to criminalize the people around them for choosing to pursue Cannabis for religious, medical, or other nonreligious purposes.

The reality is that Cannabis is literally beneficial to everyone. Cannabis can prevent disease, treat disease, and cure disease. Consuming Cannabis is a personal choice that should be a protected right for everyone. Nobody deserves to be told lies that Cannabis is poison. No religious power should be allowed to ruin someone's life for choosing Cannabis.

Here's some proof from my home state. In 2020, the state of Utah started selling medical Cannabis. In less than two years, there have been over eight hundred "Qualified Medical Providers" who have recommended and prescribed Cannabis to over fifty thousand people. Medical Cannabis has been proven to be beneficial, and there are qualified medical professionals who recommend Cannabis to everyone who is able to afford it.

New medical industries may not have the best products, they may not provide the most accurate advice, and they might be charging incredibly high prices without the option for people to homegrow Cannabis themselves. However, at least now people who can afford it are finally able to have the freedom and respect to consume Cannabis for limited medical purposes.

Yet when it comes to Cannabis, without homegrowing, we are being taken advantage of. As far as I see it, the need for Cannabis education won't end until homegrowing and consuming Cannabis become globally protected rights for the personal well-being of every individual who lives on Earth.

Cannabis consumers have a lot to consider. There are many perspectives on Cannabis out there, and you can easily run into inaccurate or incomplete sources of education. This book covers many topics that often go unspoken, but it does not provide dosage recommendations for any specific medical conditions. You must seek personal recommendations that are based on your personal medical conditions, tolerances, needs, and preferences. I believe that we all should have the protected freedom to homegrow and consume our own Cannabis. We should even have the right to sell it, assuming that local tax laws are abided by and products are able to pass local potency and contaminant testing requirements.

As we go through life, we all encounter various forms of deterioration and pain. With that in mind, Cannabis compounds are always something to consider. We are only capable of managing our personal pains and diseases according to our personal navigation of life. Many people still think that Cannabis should be avoided completely, but not everyone realizes the list of substances and illnesses that we can avoid by choosing to pursue Cannabis.

Everyone should consider themselves a candidate for Cannabis compounds. Personal religious reasons and personal allergies are the only excuses not to pursue Cannabis. However, we can no longer deny that consuming Cannabis is extremely beneficial for treating actual diseases and deteriorations throughout the body. Medical professionals can provide medical explanations as to how and why they choose to prescribe Cannabis to their patients. If someone believes psychoactive effects would not be "good" for them, well, not all compounds are psychoactive. There are Cannabis compounds that are considered nonpsychoactive, and those specific compounds can be used to benefit any targeted system in the body. Cannabis might not cure every condition completely, but it can effectively prevent, cure, and improve most pains and deteriorations people are likely to face at some point.

People of all ages and cultures have confirmed that the medical benefits of Cannabis exist, whether Cannabis is sold recreationally, medically, or even illegally. Knowledgeable medical professionals do NOT provide anti-Cannabis advice to their patients unless there is a very specific need to do so. Spreading known lies about Cannabis is manipulative, corrupt, and sometimes ignored intentionally. Once you recognize the reality of Cannabis, it becomes fairly easy to recognize that anti-Cannabis advice becomes instantly invalid the moment people begin to discredit the reality of Cannabis for those who have received guidance from medical professionals. Anti-Cannabis advice fails to consider many perspectives and ignores the big picture.

This book is a great solution for helping anyone better understand their pursuit of Cannabis. It's also a great option for medical professionals to share with any patient who might benefit by considering Cannabis for their needs.

I look forward to learning what follow-up Cannabis advice I might provide in the future, but for now, I am extremely optimistic for the potential impact of this book.

May your journey serve you well.

Consideration 1

The Many Benefits of Cannabis

We all experience pain and deterioration. So do our friends, our families, and everyone else on Earth. We all suffer individually and collectively. We might try our best to improve our personal health, but we don't always know what will provide the best benefits now and what might not be so helpful in the long run. To further complicate things, many people don't care about improving their diet or changing the substances they consume, and sometimes people who don't care about their health will teach and encourage others to do the same. Those who are deteriorating or in pain can sometimes make matters worse by consuming the wrong substances or the wrong diet. Fear mongering aside, we should all hope to improve our personal health and general well-being. It's my belief that as part of this pursuit, everyone should consider the benefits of various Cannabis compounds.

The Cannabis species contains many different compounds that can benefit any targeted system in the body. For instance, Cannabis is effective for:

- managing pain
- reducing inflammation
- promoting healthier cell death (apoptosis)
- improving digestion
- improving mental health
- enhancing nutrition (both increasing or decreasing appetite)
- reducing insomnia

These benefits exist, and we can all experience them by consuming specific Cannabis compounds. Without Cannabis, people are left to pursue these same benefits by consuming non-Cannabis substances. Keep in mind, though, just because a substance is legal, it doesn't mean that substance will be safer or less toxic than Cannabis. THC and CBD are two compounds that are commonly used to provide this list of benefits. That said, there are many other compounds out there that can provide specific benefits that THC and CBD do not.

THC and CBD have been the two most common compounds on the market for a long time, but they are not the only Cannabis compounds. The Cannabis species produces hundreds of compounds. Recommendations should be based on the research of individual Cannabis compounds. One strategy for building a recommendation is to research specific medical conditions and determine if there are specific Cannabis compounds that have been known to target or benefit those specific medical conditions. Since Cannabis isn't covered by health insurance, most of us don't have access yet to in-person recommendations from professionals who specialize in providing individualized Cannabis recommendations. This book isn't meant to provide specific recommendations for every individual, but it is meant to help you prepare for all of the different types of recommendations you might encounter. It also teaches you how to analyze, improve, or adjust any recommendation you do receive. Your pursuit of Cannabis is yours to determine, explore, and decide.

There are a lot of people out there who think they know all about Cannabis. The thing is, unless someone has years of educated experience, they probably don't know as much as they might think. In today's world, medical professionals, dedicated Cannabis advisors, and patients can all enroll in university-level Cannabis programs. We can also seek other knowledgeable professionals who might be willing to provide other suggestions for educating ourselves effectively when pursuing specific Cannabis compounds. It is beneficial to explore detailed resources on how specific conditions or systems in the body can benefit by consuming specific compounds. We cover recommendations in more detail in Consideration 4.

Becoming Knowledgeable

Personal research and exploration are critical when it comes to understanding recommendations that are designed for specific needs or preferences. Individuals have to find the right compounds, they have to be able to afford those compounds, and they must take action in consuming the right amount of compounds for their specific needs or preferences. Published experts (those who have created detailed resources, not just simplified marketing pieces designed to sell local products) can provide insight into subjects such as the specific uses for various Cannabis compounds, how to produce your own compounds by learning how to homegrow, and how to explore less-harmful consumption methods for those compounds.

There are many technical resources that can be used to research specific Cannabis compounds or how to pursue treatment for specific conditions or targeted areas in the body. Distributors and medical professionals can start helping everyone they see by directing them to educational resources that cover far more than brief conversations ever pretend to cover. Homegrowing books, online forums, local Cannabis growers, or garden supply stores can all help people who live in areas where homegrowing is permitted or where Cannabis might not be legally available for distribution.

Up-to-date resources on Cannabis compounds provide information that is far more detailed than what casual recommendations might suggest. Sharing new information with people around you and with other advisors can help improve Cannabis recommendations for others.

Beyond gaining knowledge of the various compounds, it is also helpful to learn relevant things, such as how to build tolerance for psychoactive compounds. It is also helpful to learn where to most affordably buy Cannabis compounds based on whether they are federally legal (available online and/or over the counter) or federally illegal (THC), which is commonly much more expensive. Learning to budget for different compounds can make Cannabis much more effective for anyone who is not able to afford their recommended compounds.

Cannabis compounds provide benefits to various systems in the body. Anyone providing Cannabis mentorship should know which specific compounds are best for treating targeted functions or for specific treatments. Mentorship should also include ongoing adjustments to personal tolerances and dosage requirements as needed.

Once compounds are selected for specific treatments, advisors can then decide how much and how often each compound should be recommended for specific individuals and how individuals can monitor their own consumption. For instance, if someone seems to be struggling with their tolerance when consuming psychoactive compounds, that person may benefit from reading and writing while "being high." Keeping a written journal is very effective for noticing and notating patterns of "running thoughts" when consuming THC.

One last tip for becoming knowledgeable: Find or build a community of people who are also passionate in exploring Cannabis. Cannabis book clubs, Cannabis parties, distributor events, or just meeting up with friends to discuss tips, tricks, or changes in your experience are all possibilities. Isolation can become a problem of its own with or without Cannabis. Cannabis prohibition has forced many people into isolation because they must hide themselves from people who actively choose to criminalize them for their consumption.

If you are someone who is isolated because you fear criminalization, my suggestion is to find anonymous online communities where you can openly communicate your experiences. Luckily, we live in a time where a "Cannabis Community" is just a few clicks away. If you are in isolation, be kind to yourself. Know that you are not alone. Isolation is a common defense when exploring criminalized Cannabis, but know that your pursuits are reasonable and Cannabis is providing benefits to your body. Your preferences and needs are yours to own, and you are not in the wrong for your choice to pursue Cannabis.

Benefits for Everyone

The medical benefits of Cannabis are recognized and experienced by casual consumers, patients, medical professionals, and Cannabis experts. The following list doesn't mention which compounds do what, but it does provide insight as to why Cannabis compounds are beneficial. **Each person must determine which specific compounds and dosages to consume in order to experience their own targeted benefits.** As always, ideal recommendations should include specific compounds in specific dosages based on individual needs and preferences. This list doesn't include every potential benefit of Cannabis, but here are some of the main ones:

- *Cannabis influences neurons in the body and the mind.* Working with the body's "endocannabinoid system" can be extremely effective for pain management. Endocannabinoid systems allow humans to forget or even relearn aspects and elements of pain that they manage. Relief comes when focus can be redirected from pain.
- *Cannabis provides benefits to everyone, no matter how young they are.* It is never too early to experience neurogenesis, the process of increasing neural activity throughout the brain and body. Medical professionals can prescribe Cannabis to children who are currently taking other over-the-counter or prescription medications. While some "prohibitionist experts" suspect and openly claim that neurogenesis may be harmful or dangerous to children in the long term, these claims are largely political and without substantial proof. There are many non-Cannabis alternatives supported by the medical field that are openly known to be harmful, dangerous, or even lethal to children. Consider the options.
- *Cannabis is beneficial for the elderly too.* Neurogenesis is extremely helpful in old age. Any benefit that someone can experience on this list is also beneficial to the elderly.
- *Cannabis provides aid for sleep.* Both serious and minor medical conditions can improve just by helping someone get more or better-quality sleep, especially if sleep seems to be the best way for someone to get relief from their pain. Compounds can be consumed immediately before bed to help initiate sleep or during the night to help someone fall back to sleep if needed.

- *Cannabis can provide mental distractions, personal enjoyment, and solutions for psychological pains that might otherwise be considered "inescapable" by someone.* Depression, PTSD, anger, grief, and shame are all painful experiences. These experiences may be severe, persistent, minor, or occasional. Whichever the case, recommended compounds can be used to distract the mind from an emotion or provide the opportunity to develop new patterns of thinking (neurogenesis) that have the potential to help resolve most psychological pains that may be experienced .
- *Cannabis reduces inflammation throughout the body.* This inflammation benefit is often stated lightly, but reducing inflammation is largely beneficial in helping the body recover from just being alive in general. Inflammation is increased by daily activities such as working out, overeating, and undereating as well as sickness, injury, and aging. We all require ongoing efficiencies in our body in order to reduce inflammation as much as possible.
- *Certain Cannabis compounds contribute to improved apoptosis of cells in the body.* Cells in the body are naturally designed to die off. Apoptosis encourages the natural death of cells before they generate undesirable cell mutations that can result in problematic outcomes. Some professionals recommend *flooding* the body with as many apoptosis-contributing compounds as possible. Apoptosis may not make a difference in all cases, but it can make all the difference in many cases. It is important to recognize apoptosis as a "potential medical benefit" of Cannabis, especially if "anti-cancer" effects are the intention. In some cases, Cannabis has been found to be helpful in reducing specific tumor sizes.
- *Cannabis is an effective treatment for addiction recovery.* Cannabis is a more sustainable alternative for substances such as alcohol, tobacco, sugar, meth, heroin, cocaine, prescribed pharmaceuticals, etc. It doesn't matter whether someone considers their personal consumption to be a sickness, an addiction, or a personal choice. In any case, Cannabis should be considered a valid option for replacing addictive substances, especially since alternative

substances have already been shown to provide less favorable health outcomes than beneficial Cannabis compounds.

All of the above points contribute to various forms of healing and/ or recovery for various potential medical conditions. We may not know the exact doses that are most effective for every situation, but consumers are experiencing and discovering that different compounds can be beneficial in small, medium, large, and extra-extra-extra-large doses as recommended. One thing we know for sure is that Cannabis isn't killing people at anywhere near the rate as many of the alternatives that are commonly suggested, recommended, or prescribed.

Individuals need to choose which personal recommendations to follow and navigate how much or how little Cannabis they might need or prefer. Larger doses don't always mean that additional medical benefits will be experienced, but in some cases, larger doses of specific compounds may be required in order to receive targeted benefits.

You should completely ignore the advice that Cannabis couldn't possibly medically benefit you. Cannabis is clearly medically beneficial, and we all deserve to realize that this fact is no longer debatable. While Cannabis cannot claim to heal everything, it can and does provide medical benefits to everyone who personally consumes enough of the right compounds for their specific needs or preferences. Cannabis can improve some conditions, prevent other conditions, extend life, and even promote psychological development. We can only hope for as much success as possible in determining the best treatments for each of our own preferences and medical needs.

Consideration 2

Homegrowing Is Affordable for Everyone

Currently, Cannabis dosages may cost an individual more than $10,000 in a single year. Distributors pay for labor, salaries, transportation, manufacturing, commercial licensing, taxes, rent, and other distributor-related expenses. **The solution is homegrowing.** Homegrowing removes the need to pay for commercial licensing, overpriced salaries, transportation, and taxes. Homegrowing gives us the opportunity to produce compounds for our recommendations at a fraction of the cost. Most of us will not be able to afford recommendations for Cannabis until we are allowed to homegrow our own.

Affordability is obviously an important part of the Cannabis equation. Once again, homegrowing is the solution. No one should be forced to buy high-priced products from distributors when homegrowing can provide people and families with more product than they could ever dream of affording in other markets. I believe that growing Cannabis at home should become a protected universal right for everyone in the world. Regional education is the solution for achieving legalization anywhere. Instead of Cannabis being illegal, it's the prohibition of Cannabis that should be illegal!

Every human deserves the universal right to easily afford their Cannabis recommendations by homegrowing. **If I could choose one thing for you to share with the world about this book, it would be the importance of recognizing, establishing, and protecting forever universal rights of homegrowing Cannabis for everyone.** Homegrowing for everyone is the constant battle for peace. Even if you personally decide to avoid Cannabis completely, I do hope that by reading this book, you will see why Cannabis compounds are so important to the physical and mental well-being of every living person. The benefits of Cannabis are not debatable; the benefits of Cannabis clearly exist. Not maybe, not possibly, not "we need more studies," not "not enough research"—Cannabis is beneficial, period.

Homegrowing gives the most affordable access to Cannabis. None of us should be forced to purchase high-cost products that could be homegrown. There are still billions of people out there who don't realize the major positive impacts that universal homegrowing laws would provide to everyone. We should never be forced into paying the high prices that are set by the dictated forces of other non-Cannabis-related opinions of Cannabis. Industry people have to realize that businesses are not "angel-sent" just because they sell Cannabis products. On the flip side, any person or group of people who live to legally punish, prevent, destroy, or limit Cannabis are far more destructive to humanity than ANY distributor could ever be.

Most people will never afford Cannabis without insurance coverage. Without insurance coverage, we all become financially exposed when we are faced with unaffordable access to Cannabis. Businesses are licensed to produce products, and they are able to charge their clients as much as their clients are willing to pay. The reality is that anyone can learn to homegrow Cannabis. You can grow your own Cannabis even if you are not already familiar with farming or gardening. Without homegrowing, the Cannabis community is left with getting Cannabis from various distributors, with prices that make Cannabis out of their reach.

The prohibition of homegrowing is a major financial attack on everyone who pays high prices for Cannabis products. Without homegrowing, people who consume 50mg/THC/day, or 0.25/g of 20%/THC/Flower, could end up spending between $504 and $2,520+/ year. People who consume 500mg/THC/day, or 2.5/g of 20%THC/ Flower, could end up spending between $5,040 and $25,200+/ year. For those not familiar with dosages, there are people who are recommended to consume far more than 500mg/THC/day.

All Cannabis Prohibition Is Destructive, Abusive, Corrupt, Oppressive, and Unsustainable

Cannabis prohibition should never exist. Anti-cannabis laws were established by religious teachings and beliefs of local populations. Throughout history, religious laws often have been used to recruit, attack, or destroy anyone who is caught not obeying religious rules. Democracy isn't controlled by humans; democracy is manipulated by individuals who lie and hide their involvement with corporate or religion-based agendas.

Our right to Cannabis must be pursued to the fullest extent. I believe strongly that we should globally unite in ending all drug wars IMMEDIATELY. Universally ending any prohibition of homegrowing Cannabis is an obvious reality that must be pursued for all of humankind. Cannabis is universally needed in this world. Wars involving prohibited substances have plagued this world for far too long. We should not allow anyone to criminalize anyone for their contributions to the Cannabis industry. Enough is enough. Religious manipulation of culture-controlling laws must cease to dominate those who do not share the same religious beliefs.

Sustainable and localized Cannabis is majorly important to ensuring that everyone can access Cannabis without being financially extorted for that decision. Sustainable community farming can and should be taught and encouraged by every culture and country on Earth. Our world is constantly changing, but our world will be much better off once everyone can understand the reality of what homegrowing means for all of us. Substance prohibition is war. Cannabis should be allowed, and the only war that should be fought is the one against wrongfully established Cannabis laws. It's time to free ourselves from any religious belief we do not personally choose for our own personal journey in life. Established religious laws often lead to the destruction of freedom and free will for every nonconforming human belief or action. Just because you have the freedom to think or speak about Cannabis, this does not mean you have the freedom to actually pursue Cannabis. At this point in history, continuing established religious laws is less important than protecting the reality of what Cannabis is for all of us.

Legalizing Homegrowing Makes Cannabis Affordable

Legalizing Cannabis distribution doesn't guarantee access to "affordable Cannabis"—legalizing homegrowing does. Humans deserve the right to choose Cannabis. Freedom in personal consumption and production is inevitable, natural, and should become effective immediately. None of us should be forced into paying for overpriced or overtaxed products. Homegrowing is a tool in life we all deserve. The human culture of Cannabis should not be controlled by the opinions of people who choose not to consume it. Cannabis culture should be under full control of every individual who decides to grow, consume, or distribute it. Outside cultures do not deserve payment for their manipulated involvement of the medical, spiritual, or religious beliefs of other people. Rulers do not deserve payment for their corruption of Cannabis. No religion or religious belief should be allowed to dictate the laws or culture of other religions or spiritual people who do make the conscious decision to pursue Cannabis.

Cost is a major limiting factor when making any recommendation for Cannabis consumption. If Cannabis is not affordable, people won't be aware of its benefits, and many will continue to suffer unnecessarily. The cultures of the world must unite to pursue and utilize Cannabis as a way to provide significant reductions of mass suffering throughout the world.

We've seen the harmful effects of alcohol and tobacco. To continue to promote these substances over Cannabis is damaging to everyone. We are all in this together.

This book doesn't presume to know how much Cannabis any specific person or family might need or prefer. Cannabis is a personal decision for anyone to make based on the recommendations they choose to explore. Each of us has a unique story, with unique needs and preferences. There's no way for me to know which conditions someone might already have or might be likely to encounter later in life. That said, Cannabis can and should be recommended to everyone according to their specific needs and preferences. Freedom of consumption should belong to everyone. If homegrowing is not an option, then it's not possible for everyone to realize the benefits of Cannabis and be free from suffering as they could and should be.

If you're reading this book and are unable to afford legalized Cannabis, here are some options you might consider:

- Contact your local politicians. Most politicians do not realize how low-income people will ALWAYS suffer without homegrowing protections. You can help politicians to understand that homegrowing is the solution for everyone.
- Ask local distributors if you might qualify for a reduced-pricing program for those who cannot afford their recommended dosages.
- Move to another state, or country, where Cannabis is more affordable.
- Move to another state, or country, that provides protections for homegrowing.

The way to legalization is providing the right education to the right people. When politicians and the people who vote for politicians both understand Cannabis, there will be a much greater chance of abolishing the prohibition of Cannabis. Gaining the support of all religious institutions is also of extreme importance. Without their acceptance, they will continue to control the life of nonreligious people. If people who vote are not educated, then politicians will continue to maintain criminalization of recreational, medical, spiritual, and religious use of Cannabis. Laws that prohibit or criminalize Cannabis are corrupt, ignorant, and destructive to everyone who individually chooses to pursue Cannabis for whatever purpose. Providing education to the masses is the only path to legalization. If people don't understand Cannabis, they will be subject to the understanding of others. If people in your area refuse to educate themselves, relocating may be your better option.

Useful Insights If You Are Legally Allowed to Homegrow

Growing Cannabis is similar to growing many other crops such as peppers, cucumbers, or tomatoes. Books, blogs, farmers, gardeners, and garden supply stores are all able to assist you in budgeting, growing, harvesting, and producing homegrown Cannabis products. Seed and clone distributors will often provide their customers with useful growing information such as which compounds the plant has been shown to produce (psychoactive or nonpsychoactive), length of time for flowering, range estimates for expected yields, and optimal environmental conditions for growth.

People can homegrow for their needs and preferences, and they can also grow additional plants for the needs and preferences of family and friends who cannot afford to pursue Cannabis. In one harvest, one single Cannabis plant could produce as little as one ounce of flower, or it could produce more than ten pounds of flower. Harvest totals are determined by grower skills, environmental growing conditions, and the genetic potential of each plant.

Seeds and clones don't contain any THC. When it comes to shipping seeds and clones, plants don't produce THC until they begin their "flowering cycle." Note: Since there is no THC present, many seed and clone distributors are willing to ship their genetics to most places in the world. However, just because it is legal for distributors to send seeds or clones, this does not mean those seeds or clones will be legal to homegrow.

Growing Cannabis at home is an exciting and rewarding endeavor that can enhance your life in both expected and unexpected ways. I hope you will explore this for yourself and join the ranks of those who benefit from homegrowing.

Consideration 3

Distribution Industries, and the Need to End All Drug Wars

Just because we are allowed to buy Cannabis doesn't mean we will be able to afford the recommended dosages. Most of us don't realize that we should consider Cannabis if we find ourselves in pain, having sleeping problems, require specific treatments, or are consuming other substances that have proven to be more harmful than Cannabis.

Those of us who have always had access to Cannabis often forget that there are still entire countries in this world where people just like us are criminalized for any involvement in Cannabis. If people cannot afford as much Cannabis as they desire or require, then their access to Cannabis does not actually exist. Homegrowing makes Cannabis affordable and accessible to everyone. Eventually, humans will realize how important our freedom is and why our freedom does not exist without universal homegrowing protections for every person.

The Types of Cannabis Distribution:

1. **Recreational Distribution**
2. **Medical Distribution**
3. **Criminalized Distribution**

Recreational Distribution

Recreational states allow adults over the age of twenty-one to purchase Cannabis. This seems reasonable, until one realizes that recreational pricing is still not determined according to what most people are able to afford. Government institutions, hidden agendas buried in religious laws, and money-oriented corporations are all aimed at capturing as much money from the Cannabis community as possible. If homegrowing is not allowed, affordable Cannabis will not be accessible to everyone.

The good thing about recreational industries is that adults aren't required to justify their consumption to medical field experts when they aren't looking for "help." Recreational industries don't require adults to justify, explain, or pay for medical recommendations. Recreational industries allow people who are "old enough" to buy products from the corporations that the state sells licenses to. People who consume Cannabis are usually not covered or protected by their medical insurance. Without access to legalized homegrowing, the Cannabis community is left facing prices that are much higher than what could be produced in their own homes.

Medical Distribution

Like recreational industries, medical industries also require product testing for contaminants and potency. However, people are required to justify, document, and pay medical professionals in order to receive recommendations or purchase medical Cannabis. Medical industries allow some people to afford Cannabis, but most people are left without proper guidance or financial support from medical Cannabis industries.

Some medical industries require "medical pharmacies" to hire state-licensed pharmacists to "approve" each transaction. The micro-oversight of requiring a medical pharmacist to regulate Cannabis distribution is unhelpful to everyone. Nobody should be forced to pay for the expensive distribution requirements of professionals providing an unneeded service. Drug pharmacists hold degrees so they can distribute "pharmacy drugs" that are often more harmful or even deadly if dosages are miscalculated. Providing Cannabis to people does not and should not require a college-level education. Why? Because Cannabis is beneficial and not casually deadly to consumers. Micromanaged services should not be allowed to be required if insurance is unable to be accepted for required services. Medical professionals should not be allowed to profit from Cannabis recommendations if they are unable to bill insurance companies or provide a service that is actually needed or specialized. Just because pharmacists are "required" does NOT mean they are experts in regard to Cannabis.

Whether medical professionals profit or not, we should all be encouraged to pursue Cannabis because of how beneficial it is for every system in the body. We shouldn't be sold other drugs just because a medical professional can't get a vacation or paycheck from their friendly neighborhood drug representative as compensation. We all deserve to have protected universal rights to homegrowing Cannabis.

If medical professionals are not experts in Cannabis, while positioning their advice as "expert-level advice," they should preface their recommendations by telling people that their medical degrees do not make them experts in Cannabis. People who think medical professionals are the right experts to trust probably don't realize that many medical professionals aren't properly educated in Cannabis. There is an obvious problem when medical professionals are not providing accurate Cannabis compound recommendations for specifically targeted treatments. All in all, medical professionals should be suggesting Cannabis, not selling everyone other drugs just because they aren't allowed to suggest Cannabis. They also shouldn't be required to provide recommendations if insurance is unable to cover the cost to fill prescriptions or receive recommendations for Cannabis.

Until federal legalization takes place, insurance companies will be forced to ignore the needs of everyone who chooses to consume Cannabis. Most of us could benefit by receiving medical oversight throughout their navigation of Cannabis, but people who do not require assistance should not be required to buy into the advice of medical professionals who aren't providing accurate or sufficient Cannabis education to literally anyone.

The problem with the medical industry "running Cannabis" is that there are too many people (literally everyone) for medical professionals to effectively teach and recommend Cannabis to.

Advisors should be providing or suggesting educated resources; not attempting fifteen-minute conversations to help someone completely understand Cannabis. Medical professionals shouldn't advise their patients about Cannabis unless they are willing to become actual experts on Cannabis. There is more to consider than just the fact that smoking flower is worse than vaping flower or concentrates. At this point, there are not enough medical professionals to appropriately manage every single person's recommendation for Cannabis. Modern educational resources should be recommending Cannabis to everyone.

Medical professionals have other jobs to do besides charge everyone they see for ongoing recommendations for Cannabis. Medical professionals shouldn't be charging for Cannabis advice if they are not providing expert-level recommendations or extensive and effective education to their patients.

Everyone deserves to know that Cannabis is medically beneficial, but they should also realize that medical professionals are not always the best experts to give Cannabis recommendations. Medical professionals are only allowed to prescribe Cannabis if it is legal where they are employed, and they are putting their medical degrees at risk if they do not provide the advice they are instructed to provide. Professionals cannot properly teach or recommend Cannabis to anyone if they are not actual experts in Cannabis.

Charging everyone for advice regarding general health is one thing. If medical professionals are not properly educating people on Cannabis, they end up putting everyone they talk to at risk by providing inaccurate or incomplete recommendations for Cannabis. Bad or incomplete advice can lead people to overpaying, failing, or even quitting Cannabis completely.

Only some people will need specific instructions on how to use and enjoy the Cannabis compounds they are recommended to consume. Some people prefer to consume very little psychoactive compounds, while others might need or prefer well over 500mg/THC/day. People need more than to be told to beware of psychoactive effects and to consume the least amount of Cannabis compounds as possible. This common example of non-advice does and will be likely to lead people to failing in their pursuit of Cannabis. This in turn leads them right back toward consuming less-beneficial alternatives. If erroneous guidance is provided, they can turn elsewhere for actual Cannabis advice. Cannabis experts do not provide non-Cannabis advice. There are VERY few exceptions.

Medical industries have developed specific guidelines for the treatments they provide and recommend to everyone. Medical industries are not allowed to include Cannabis alongside other suggestions in cases where Cannabis isn't legalized medically. If Cannabis were legalized, then medical guidelines could integrate Cannabis compound treatments into their other extensive treatment options. Many medical professionals are only allowed to vaguely suggest that other people have mentioned having success by consuming Cannabis. They may not be able to provide advice as to which specific compounds will provide the most benefits for specifically targeted treatments. The answer is to look for medical professionals who are capable of providing expert-level advice.

Criminalized Distribution

Anti-Cannabis laws do not allow legal distribution. Not all illegal products are tested for contaminants or purity. Lab testing is available to those who want to send their Cannabis products to a lab for testing, but some choose to blindly trust their own judgment as to whether products are worth the price they pay or not. Personal judgment does not ensure that products will be free from contaminants. Lab testing is the only way to truly ensure that any product is clean, and that is exactly why all products require testing before they are able to be sold to the public. Some criminalized distributors hold themselves to a high standard and ensure their products undergo adequate testing, but for the most part, the majority of unregulated Cannabis is untested. That said, why shouldn't homegrowers be allowed to sell products that are lab-tested while other commercially licensed growers can legally profit from multiple acres of year-round greenhouse production?

Illegal markets continue to incriminate anyone caught possessing or consuming Cannabis—from everyone who consumes it and medical professionals to growers and distributors. It's not about who isn't willing to pay taxes, it's about laws not allowing people to obtain business licenses so they can legally pay taxes on the work they do.

Illegal markets perpetuate the empowerment of racism by empowering individuals to personally criminalize any person not obeying laws that they "personally support." Cannabis consumers are unjustly discriminated against, and corrupt corporations are designed to profit from the criminalization of innocent people. Military and any other emergency responders deserve to be given their rightful freedom to consume Cannabis as well. **Not allowing humans to consume Cannabis is more of a crime against humankind than any amount of illegal distribution.**

The misguided prohibition of Cannabis, and suppression of its culture, is the exact opposite of public safety. Nobody deserves to be misguided toward commonly consumed substances that knowingly cause more harm than Cannabis due to the uninformed opinion or misleading agendas of others. Cannabis prohibition continues to be harmful to everyone who continues thinking that Cannabis is dangerous and should not ever be considered unless "absolutely necessary." In my opinion, Cannabis prohibition, along with any other war on drugs, is the largest root of all corruption and suffering that exist in this world.

People alive during Cannabis prohibition should be provided with free legal Cannabis licenses and *prohibition reparation tax deductions* whether they continue working within the Cannabis industry or not. Tax deductions equal to time lost, abuse to peace of mind, and money lost by Cannabis industry workers who have been criminalized and corruptly removed from their "medical industry" of choice during and despite the prohibition of others.

We must end prohibition efforts worldwide for the personal freedom of all future generations. Homegrowing and equally regulated trade must become the global standard for Cannabis policy. Local production of all substances should be the ultimate goal for every modern civilization. We can work together to create a world with more accessible abundance for everyone. In fact, we must if we ever expect to provide adequate food, water, substances, and housing as sustainably as possible.

The Rights for Homegrowing Cannabis Must Be Protected Forever

"Let freedom ring," but only if the people choose it. Until we are able to choose freedom, we will be actively promoting and distributing far less beneficial substances to cultures of people who are experiencing painful lifestyles. At this point, the corruption is clear, obvious, and must become common knowledge until all wars on drugs are ended throughout the entire world for all of us. We have to put an end to all drug criminalization that continues to prey on the labors and lives of hardworking people. In particular, the war against Cannabis must end globally. Humanity must choose to end war.

Everyone should have the equal right to cultivate Cannabis and pay taxes on lab-tested products that are sold. We should all have the right to produce, consume, and distribute any substance that humans choose to pursue. Modern civilization is too massive to continue running on globally distributed substances. If we want a more sustainable world, we need to learn how to create sustainable abundance everywhere. All humans NEED all-season greenhouses, sustainable water conservation, and shelters made from locally sourced materials. Cannabis can be used sustainably to create pretty much ANYTHING.

Cannabis is not considered a "protected class" in the United States, although there have been places within the United States where people can no longer be fired for "off the clock" consumption of Cannabis. It's a step in the right direction, but we should also have the freedom and respect to consume Cannabis whenever we choose to do so.

Since Cannabis is not a protected class, people who consume Cannabis can be legally discriminated against when Cannabis prohibition laws are broken. Cannabis consumers, patients, medical professionals, or spiritual leaders legally can be fired, have their children taken from them, be evicted, fined, and criminally prosecuted in court. By legal definition, people are allowed to be enslaved, be put in jail or in prison if they are caught consuming or possessing Cannabis.

Consuming Cannabis should not be prohibited and made punishable due to religious oppression. This situation has been created by certain organizations that seek to impose an "all-righteous" reality ever since their finances have been tax-exempt and used to maintain cultural "standards" through misguided manipulations of the public. MAN-MADE FALSE RIGHTEOUSNESS will never prevail against the UNIVERSAL TRUTH that is the free agency of every human soul. Cannabis will continue to decrease suffering on Earth. The internet of human communication must stop allowing false "righteousness laws" to dictate our shared existence.

No war is a war worth having when peace, freedom, and localized abundance are possible solutions. All drugs must be allowed in order for all wars to end. Any single act of criminalization of any drug perpetuates the destructive domination of "other human beings." Drug and food production should both be pursued as sustainably as possible. The choice to grow or produce any substance should be universally protected, and local environments should recognize that any attempt to interfere with the freedom of others is an obvious sign of corruption. Outsourcing substances forces people into living dangerously while engaging with networks of criminalized individuals who are considered to be "at war" with the many legal organizations that are designed to collect as much profit as possible from the Cannabis community.

All drug wars must end. I am calling this out into the world now so all nations will be forced to articulate to "their humans" why their involvement in drug wars must continue and why "their humans" will not be receiving free agency in their lifetime. We must give peace a chance.

My soul cannot and will not be ruled by corrupt dictators. Ending all war should always be a dream humans chase, and it can only start by ending all war on drugs for the purpose of restoring free agency and freedom to all local communities who could then provide their own abundances by producing their own localized food or substances.

Upholding our communities is more important than upholding the beliefs that have worked so hard to cover and destroy the reality of what Cannabis is. We will always deserve our human right to free agency in homegrowing any chosen compound.

Consideration 4

What Common Cannabis Advice Looks Like— And What It Should Look Like

Throughout history, people have debated whether Cannabis was beneficial or not. Today, there are no stable arguments proving that Cannabis is not beneficial to everyone. Cannabis compounds are beneficial in many regards. Certain people's opinions may never change, but the industry of Cannabis will continue to expand globally because recommendations, education, legal rights, and products will continue to innovate as time continues. Everyone should have freedom to choose Cannabis.

There are more than 8 billion people on Earth. Every person has their own understanding of Cannabis, and today humans are able to fact-check information unlike any other time in history. Not everyone has the same type of understanding of Cannabis, but misinformation is becoming easier and easier to debunk with online research. When it comes to Cannabis, there are still millions of people around the world who don't realize that their knowledge of Cannabis may be outdated.

Many common thoughts on Cannabis may have sounded reasonable in conversation before smartphones but eventually have turned out to be factually incorrect. There are still billions of people who incorrectly imagine concepts such as:

- Nonpsychoactive compounds are best because "feeling different" should be avoided.

- Nonpsychoactive compounds provide the same benefits as psychoactive compounds.
- Psychoactive compounds are best, and nonpsychoactive compounds are not beneficial.
- There are no beneficial Cannabis compounds for anyone.

The fact is that everyone should prepare themselves for consuming both psychoactive and nonpsychoactive Cannabis compounds because they are beneficial to many functions of the body. Avoiding psychoactive compounds completely may be preferred, but there are times when psychoactive compounds are the recommended solution for targeting specific receptors in the body. Starting recommendations can range from small doses to large doses, but most people should expect that eventually high dosages could be recommended as treatment for a large variety of deteriorating bodily conditions.

If someone doesn't "feel ready" to consume psychoactive Cannabis compounds when they are needed, then they may be likely to accept suggestions for other potential substances for treatment. Cannabis has been shown to be more beneficial and less dangerous than many other substances that are commonly recommended and regularly suggested to consumers of all ages.

CBD and THC are the most commonly recommended compounds. CBD is nonpsychoactive and can be used to treat pain and provide other helpful advantages to the body. There are many other beneficial compounds that are also nonpsychoactive. Meanwhile, THC is psychoactive and can provide a completely different set of advantages to the body. There are also many other beneficial compounds that are psychoactive.

Various experts have already answered the question: "Should Cannabis be recommended to everyone?" The short answer is: "Yes, it should." Modern experts are far more likely to be asking questions such as:

- "How much do individuals prefer recreationally?"
- "How much might someone medically require for desired treatment results?"

- "Which products are best?"
- "When is the best time to consume specific compounds?"
- "What are the most affordable ways for people to access the Cannabis compounds they are recommended to consume in their local area?"

If people don't have solutions for potential questions like these, they are missing many relevant details in regards to their own personal pursuit of Cannabis .

Without adequate Cannabis education, people are far more likely to pursue casual suggestions or professional recommendations for other less beneficial substances. People tend to pursue advice from people they trust. These might include trusted friends, family members, religious mentors, product distributors, service providers and medical professionals. Many available substances would never be recommended by Cannabis-educated experts who provide detailed suggestions and recommendations for Cannabis to every person they encounter.

Expert-level recommendations should include as many of these details as possible:

1. Which compounds to use for specific treatments
2. Suggested size, frequency, and timing for psychoactive treatments
3. Suggested size, frequency, and timing for nonpsychoactive treatments
4. How much of each compound to consume per dose/per day/per month/per year(s)
5. Which products to buy and where to buy them
6. What to expect when consuming and dosing various types of products
7. How to plan for legal homegrowing if personal financing is low or nonexistent
8. Knowing when to determine whether adjustments are either needed or preferred

You can find expert-level Cannabis advice online, and you can contact various Cannabis advisory services by phone. It's important to compare different sources until you feel confident that the planned dosages are the best according to your specific medical needs or recreational preferences. Anyone receiving advice chooses whether to act based on that advice or continue their search for better-suited advice. Fortunately, we can quickly fact-check most questions by researching multiple online resources and comparing all recommendations before making a personal decision to ever consume anything. If someone isn't willing to recommend Cannabis compounds to their own family, then what substances will their families be likely to consume?

People who are most familiar with Cannabis regularly recommend specific compounds because they understand how and why compounds are beneficial to different systems in the body. Cannabis does what it does whether someone understands the reality of how it affects the body or not. Cannabis experts understand how to adjust recommendations according to the needs and preferences whenever they are providing recommendations while also teaching people to make their own adjustments and best navigate their local laws and available pricing based on their specific environmental conditions.

We usually get advice from people we trust (friends, family, mentors), distributors, and medical professionals. We should always consider the educational background of anyone providing recommendations and whether or not that person is in fact familiar and educated in Cannabis. Most of us don't have Cannabis experts in our immediate circle of people we trust. This book is meant to help you to be more confident and knowledgeable when deciding whose recommendations to live by.

Not Everybody Who Talks About Cannabis Actually Knows What They Are Talking About

You should always take advice with caution. If someone giving Cannabis advice doesn't teach or provide good resources on topics such as vaporization versus combustion, nano-emulsions, apoptosis, or solventless extraction, then they are not providing expert-level education to anyone. *Giving partial advice* and *providing adequate education* are two very different levels of service.

Trusted advisors are friends, family, and mentors whom you trust. Not all trusted advisors are experienced or educated when it comes to Cannabis. Therefore, not all trusted advisors are capable of providing accurate recommendations for Cannabis. There are advisors who persuade people to avoid Cannabis because they do not think Cannabis is beneficial. Whether they realize it or not, those advisors are failing to acknowledge the literal benefits that many people experience every single day. Cannabis compounds can be beneficial to any targeted system in the body.

People who are not sharing accurate information on Cannabis don't realize how dangerous their advice might actually become for someone. Advisors who fail to acknowledge the many realities of Cannabis are providing a major disservice to every person who trusts them to provide as many benefits as possible. If someone isn't thoroughly educated in Cannabis, they won't be capable of providing the best recommendations possible today.

Non-Cannabis recommendations rarely come from actual experts of Cannabis. Non-Cannabis recommendations assume that there are no medical benefits to consuming Cannabis and that everyone is better off using either non-Cannabis alternatives or nothing at all. Non-Cannabis advice is provided by people who are either intentionally or accidentally undereducated in the commonly documented benefits of Cannabis. Not recommending Cannabis is dangerous advice to give. If someone doesn't recommend Cannabis, what might they suggest for replacing the benefits of Cannabis?

Not all recommendations are perfect. Just because someone has the ability to provide expert-level recommendations doesn't mean they will or have always effectively delivered their expert-level knowledge. Education can be made simple to help people get started, but Cannabis is not simple, and people shouldn't be under the impression that it is. Simplified education should be accompanied with other expert-level resources that support the simplified education of any products that are sold. If expert-level resources are not made available, suggestions for expert-level resources should be provided and mentioned every time a product is sold.

There are a lot of excellent advocates out there who are able to answer the questions and concerns that most people tend to ask. Advocates may be impactful in convincing people to try Cannabis, but incomplete or inaccurate advice can lead to people missing many important considerations. There are people who will not succeed in Cannabis without receiving expert-level, step-by-step guidance for their specific treatments. Incomplete advice fails to address questions people simply don't realize they should be asking. Providing accurate educational resources is the only way to ensure that people have all the information they need or want to consider in any personal pursuit of Cannabis.

If you are not familiar with Cannabis, don't expect to learn it from someone who is unable to provide expert-level education, expert-level resources, or expert-level recommendations. If someone does not recommend Cannabis, it's because they are unable to do so.

Distributors Should Focus on Sharing Expert-Level Resources

Most people end up getting some sort of advice from their distributor. Distributors include dispensaries (recreational adult use), street dealers (criminalized Cannabis), and Cannabis pharmacies (medical use). Selling Cannabis does not automatically mean someone is an expert-level Cannabis educator. Providing quality lab-tested products is a helpful service, but not all distributors recommend expert-level educational resources to their clients. Non-experts of Cannabis are not capable of providing enough relevant consideration during brief or casual conversation. Even Cannabis experts should consider moments when they too have delivered partial or inadequate education.

Many distributors are able to answer most questions their clients ask, but they may not know how to create or suggest comprehensive expert-level education. Some distributors have created incredible educational content for their clients, but education is almost always missing details on many important Cannabis topics. For instance, expert-level education shouldn't leave people chasing Sativa head highs and Indica body highs for treatments.

There are many relevant Cannabis topics people should be educated on. However, just because a distributor offers simplified education that looks good or sounds good to people doesn't make it good education in the short term or long term. Education is typically centered around products offered instead of teaching people that homegrowing might be their most affordable option for accessing Cannabis compounds. Instead of sharing the best possible insight in a given moment, educators should reflect on past conversations and consider whether providing long-term resources might have been better than providing quick advice.

If experts do not create their own expert-level education, they should be sharing other expert-level educational resources with everyone they can. Simplified education doesn't teach Cannabis to people; it only introduces them to that specific explanation of Cannabis. There is a major difference. Simplified education can be found everywhere, while expert-level education is extremely rare in comparison. The only thing missing is that people who are only providing simplified education should be helping people locate resources that provide a more in-depth perspective of the recommendations and products they might provide.

Quick product education is helpful when people don't know what they are looking at, but everyone should consider many other educational topics as well. Cannabis is not simple just because someone thinks they figured out an easy way to explain something. Cannabis is complex and people need to recognize this so they don't pursue Cannabis based on other inaccurate or oversimplified education that might be missing relevant topics.

Cannabis Advice from Medical Professionals

Medical professionals often work extremely long hours and are constantly meeting with people who will either need or prefer specific treatments. Medical professionals may have years of schooling, but if they do not pursue expert-level Cannabis education, they may have a hard time providing expert-level education or recommendations to anyone. Cannabis education isn't as simple as giving someone a quick mention that they should definitely consume Cannabis. Cannabis education should include both expert-level education and guided recommendations for each person. We need guidance in understanding how and why we should pursue Cannabis and how to become as successful as possible in that pursuit.

Most medical professionals are rightfully hesitant to prescribe a Schedule 1 substance that could put their career and/or medical degrees at risk. This is understandable, but it leads many people to consume other less beneficial recommendations. Many medical professionals have no problems comprehending why that is true. If medical professionals are allowed to recommend Cannabis, they should learn which expert-level educational resources they can recommend to everyone. Simple or casual education often leaves people still feeling the need to find actual educational resources of their own.

More and more medical professionals are learning to improve their recommendations of Cannabis. States with medical Cannabis programs do provide simplified education to their licensed medical professionals. However, simplified "medical education" doesn't magically turn medical professionals into Cannabis experts. This type of education creates medical professionals who are allowed to prescribe Cannabis even if they are not capable of providing expert-level Cannabis education or recommendations to anyone.

Incomplete recommendations and simplified education do not properly prepare people for Cannabis. Undereducated professionals who provide recommendations in the industry should know which expert-level resources they like to recommend to individuals with various conditions, needs, or preferences. After reading this book, medical professionals should realize how they can either develop their own version of expert-level recommendations or suggest other expert-level resources. Medical professionals shouldn't leave people without expert-level recommendations or expert-level educational resources. Simplified education is far better than anti-Cannabis advice, but simplified education should be replaced with expert-level recommendations or expert-level educational resources.

There is another giant problem with medical professionals recommending Cannabis today. Without insurance coverage, medical professionals don't have much choice but to continue writing other drug prescriptions to people who are not allowed to homegrow and have no way to afford medical or recreational distributor prices. People should always keep an eye out for who is genuinely trying to help them and who is trying to get them to pay "top-shelf pricing" for Cannabis that doesn't even come close to the best quality.

Those who are able to develop expert-level recommendations will be able to provide better recommendations for Cannabis than medical professionals who are not experts in Cannabis. That said, this book should inspire many medical professionals to explore other expert-level resources. Medical professionals will need to seek other resources and/or textbooks that can provide suggested recommendations of specific Cannabis compounds for specific treatments.

This book is meant to provide an incredible starting point for any medical professional interested in becoming an actual expert in Cannabis. This book may not make an instant expert out of every medical professional, but I am confident that it does point both medical professionals and any other reader in the right direction.

This book should lead people to creating recommendations that are better than what other non-experts of Cannabis will be likely to offer. This book goes beyond just casually mentioning that Cannabis is for everyone. My goal is to teach people how to understand Cannabis to the very best of my ability. Writing books is an art, and art is a difficult place to achieve perfection, but I think this is about as close as I could get without attempting to provide actual compound recommendations for every situation I could possibly think of.

We all must trust our own judgment and determine which recommendations we will choose to pursue. You should always mention any concerns or suggestions you recognize when receiving any recommendation. This is not for the purpose of arguing, but for the purpose of learning how a recommendation might be improved through further consideration. If anyone is able to improve an advisor's knowledge of Cannabis, then that advisor should be able to provide improved recommendations.

Selling medical services without providing expert-level education or insurance coverage leads many people to fail in their pursuit of enjoying or benefiting from Cannabis. For example, a person's recommendation may be reduced because they can only afford a certain amount of compounds for their dosages. Recommendations should not just be blindly reduced. Small dosages are not as helpful if large doses are needed for proper treatment. If dosage sizes are unaffordable, then real experts should be educating those people on the steps they can or should take in order to best afford their actual recommended dosages.

For clarification, this section is meant to educate you on noticing that non-Cannabis advice is not the opinion of Cannabis experts, how to spot expert-level recommendations, and to help you realize that not all simplified education should be considered expert-level education. Only an actual Cannabis expert will be able to provide actual expert-level education or recommendations.

Consideration 5

Strain Labels, Product Labels, and the Art of Navigating Psychoactive Compounds

People have been categorizing Cannabis long before we learned to produce isolated compounds. Indica, Sativa, Ruderalis (Autos), and Hybrid are four names that have been largely used to categorize the different origins and characteristics of different strains of Cannabis. These four categories are known as *strain labels*. Strain labels have been used to describe the effects of different Cannabis strains. Knowing about strain labels can be useful for plant breeding or when the compounds of a strain are completely unknown without seeking detailed lab results for specific compounds. **In other words, strain labels do not tell buyers which compounds they are actually buying.** It is important to realize that treatment recommendations can be used to pursue expected effects, but recommendations for specific ratios of Cannabis compounds might, and very well could be, the more suitable recommendation to share with everyone.

I used to love to share the classic lines: "Indica: in-da-couch; Sativa: head high; and Hybrid: body and head high. Head high and body high seemed to fit when describing certain strains. What I didn't realize was that these strain labels were also used to classify Cannabis based on a strain's country of origin or how a plant might look while it is growing. Today, I've come to the conclusion that people are much better off pursuing specific Cannabis compounds than the effects of strain labels. Teaching people to make purchases based on strain labels may or may not lead them to understanding their preferences or needs for specific compounds. Allow me to elaborate.

Why Product Labels Should Be Used Before Relying on Strain Labels

Most Cannabis buyers end up shopping for products that will provide them with as many recommended compounds as they can possibly afford. This is especially true if they are not covered by medical insurance or not allowed to homegrow their own Cannabis. Be aware that not all medical professionals in your area will be capable of providing expert-level Cannabis recommendations. You can always refer back to Consideration 4 if you don't remember what expert-level recommendations should look like.

Also see Consideration 8 for more details on sourcing various compounds. Some people might not receive the benefits they are expecting if they do not pursue expert-level recommendations first. We don't receive every possible benefit of Cannabis just because we consume it. Casual education only goes so far when it comes to refining and tailoring specific recommendations for people who are often hoping or praying to receive as many benefits from Cannabis as possible.

Strain labels have been used to describe various characteristics of Cannabis, such as geographic origins, physical plant characteristics, and expected strain effects. Strain labels are not based on the specific compounds found in a strain. The genomic mapping of many Cannabis species is proof that strain labels don't always guarantee the same Cannabis compounds or the same estimated effects. Each strain label was "invented" by completely different people sometime between 1548 and 1930. In fact, strain labels were created long before we had even discovered various compounds such as CBN (1940), CBD (1942), or THC (1964). Long before strain labels, the first-known Cannabis ever mentioned in medicinal texts was titled "Ma" in 2700 BCE China. Over 4,720 years ago humans mentioned that

Cannabis could be consumed. Cannabis has been around for a long time.

Strain labels can help experienced consumers choose strains according to perceived preferences, but even experienced consumers should read "product labels" first. Product labels should include the total mg amounts for each Cannabis compound found in a product. Making purchases based on estimated strain effects may be misleading if someone doesn't have recommendations for specific compounds for their treatment. Those who have specific dosage recommendations should seek out those specific compounds. Once we know that we're buying the right compounds for our preferences and needs, we can start to consider which strain labels we prefer over others.

So, while strain labels are still used today, we now know that those terms are not based on which compounds are present. So yes, these labels do exist, but we now know that we should be looking for specific Cannabis compounds for treatment instead of guessing the contents or effects that a strain may or may not actually contain.

We should only be concerned with strain labels if a product label is not provided. Even without a label, we can still research the name of a strain (if it is known) to learn which compounds the strain will be likely to contain. Knowing whether something is an Indica or a Sativa does not dictate which compounds will be found in the strain.

Not all Sativas produce the same compounds; not all Indicas produce the same compounds; not all Ruderalis produce the same compounds; not all Hybrids produce the same compounds. Whether we need or prefer to consume specific compounds, only products that contain labels will list the compounds that are contained within a product.

We should seek to know which compounds we need or prefer and which products we will need to buy. We should not just expect to feel the effects that a strain label might lead us to assume. Again, strain labels can be helpful, but we should pursue specific education on which Cannabis compounds provide specific benefits before going strain hunting for specific effects.

An Overview of Compounds and the Oversimplified Use of Strain Labels

Cannabis breeders technically produce new genetic crosses every time two plants pollinate and reproduce seed. Different genetic crossings have the potential to create different combinations of Cannabis compounds. Today, there are thousands of Cannabis "crosses" that have produced over 350 compounds. In order to grow all 350 compounds, a grower/breeder/cultivator might need to grow hundreds of different Cannabis species to extract every potential compound in Cannabis. Even then, many compounds have only been produced in such small trace amounts that it would require time to develop new genetic breeding, plant selection, and growing strategies just to produce them in high enough concentrations to actually create products.

Not so long ago, THC was only found in trace amounts (less than 5 percent) in most places around the world. Civilizations learned to increase THC concentrations after developing new breeding methods, plant selection, and growing strategies. Without increased potency, farmers would need to use far more water and nutrients to produce the same amount of compounds.

The same goes for CBD, CBG, and other Cannabis compounds that modern civilization has learned to produce in increasingly higher potencies. Cannabis compounds were not farmed, extracted, measured, and labeled for millions of people the way they are today. Our modern product labels were not available to consumers in the past, and we know more about specific Cannabis compounds than ever before. The era of Cannabis is here now more than ever.

Compounds are not more or less helpful to everyone just because they are more popular, affordable, or available. Every compound has its own recommended dosages. We need to explore which compounds are recommended for our specific treatment(s) based on the most current information we can possibly find. The more those who pursue Cannabis are able to learn, the more prepared everyone can be when determining which recommendations to follow. There are quite a few textbook options that provide details on specific Cannabis compounds, and many of these can be purchased online.

Anyone can use the internet to research a breeder or brand's description of the effects of a new strain they have created. Some descriptions can get pretty elaborate or accurate. However, there is no way to know how many of which compounds are inside any product without product labels detailing compound totals from lab results.

Sometimes, previous lab results will be provided in a strain's description. Strain descriptions may be helpful if no product labels are provided and all someone can do is guess at which compounds they are actually buying. Keep in mind that every individual plant can produce varied amounts of Cannabis compounds based on how it is grown. This means that just because a strain has had good lab results in the past, it does not mean that every crop will produce those same yields or cleanliness. Cannabis products require carefully planned testing procedures to ensure that product labels are as accurate as possible for every crop and product that is produced for sale.

Compound levels can vary from plant to plant or crop to crop. Crops grown from seed tend to have more variance in total compounds from plant to plant. Crops produced from cloning will produce less variance in total compounds because clones are more similar to the mother plants they are taken from. That is why product labels are created for every batch of product that is made. Lab testing is the only way for anyone to know exactly how much of each compound they will find in a product.

The strain labels of Indica, Sativa, Ruderalis, and Hybrid might not tell us which compounds are in a strain, but they can provide estimates as to what someone might expect to experience based on somebody else's previous experience. Once we ensure we are purchasing the specific compounds for our recommended treatments, then we can start shopping according to strain preferences. In time, consumers can learn their strain preferences for specific occasions such as working, creating, socializing, cleaning, sleeping, eating, and relaxing.

The strain labels are roughly based on these classic descriptions. Indica strains MIGHT leave some people "in da' couch" with relaxing body effects. Sativa strains MIGHT provide people with more of a cerebral or "heady" experience. Hybrids MIGHT include balanced effects of each or lean closer toward a body or a head high. Ruderalis strains go into flower faster than other strains and are often used to create shorter growth cycles when crossed with other strains that normally take much longer to harvest flower. Pure Ruderalis strains are rarely grown on their own because they do not produce as many compounds as other Indica, Sativa, or Hybrid strains that have been genetically selected for their ability to produce high compound yields.

Each strain MIGHT make someone feel more tired or awake depending on their mood, body composition, diet, sleep, and their familiarity with psychoactive effects. Strain effects do have differences, but learning to enjoy any strain can help us recognize that Cannabis isn't just about making someone feel a very specific type of way for all of time. Sometimes the pursuit of Cannabis is more about getting the right compounds in the body for specially targeted benefits and learning to enjoy that process as much as possible. In other words, we shouldn't be so insistent on specific strain types because strain types might not contain the compounds that are actually recommended for specific treatments anyway.

Preparation for Consuming Psychoactive Compounds

Exploring psychoactive compounds, such as THC in all its various forms, doesn't have to be as terrifying as you might think. Some people are recommended to take large doses of THC for specifically targeted treatment, but not everyone has the need or desire to start with large doses without practice first. That said, everyone should learn to handle large doses. Eventually, everyone reaches a point where large doses of THC may be needed. The goal should be to prefer the effects of Cannabis so that the body can have what it needs when it needs it.

Stories of "terrifying Cannabis moments" are common, but Cannabis is rarely the accurate culprit to blame. People love to blame Cannabis. People have been known to claim that Cannabis makes them totally dysfunctional or unable to focus. Some people imagine that Cannabis could never possibly be good for them. People don't always realize that claims against Cannabis are usually descriptions for their own thoughts and behaviors. They might not realize that stories of people not being able to handle Cannabis are poor descriptions for describing the reality of how Cannabis actually interacts with the body and mind. Stories and actions are created by people. Cannabis doesn't force people to create actions or stories. People do.

The Art of Navigating Psychoactive Thoughts

The human body contains neuron receptors throughout the entire body. These receptors are how our body communicates with itself. Our thoughts, our subconscious, every movement we make, and most functions in our body are all functions that involve our neuron receptors. Our receptors are affected by everything we consume. Every substance we consume has different effects on our neuron receptors. Every substance we consume also affects our internal organs differently. Cannabis compounds don't have the same effects on our internal organs that many other regularly consumed substances do.

People are likely to encounter various "trains of thought" when their neurons are affected by THC. These "trains of thought" exist with or without Cannabis. The difference is that these two "trains of thought" might seem more intense, inescapable, noticeable or out of the ordinary if someone takes more Cannabis than they are comfortable with.

The two main "trains of thought" to look out for are hyperfocusing thoughts and racing thoughts. Hyperfocusing and racing thoughts might seem simple, but increased neuron activity can become extremely overwhelming when someone is not properly prepared to tolerate longer durations of psychoactive activity. Recognizing these two potentials will be very useful while learning to navigate psychoactive activity.

People can learn to catch themselves hyperfocusing and choose whether specific thoughts are something they actually want to be hyperfocusing on or not. They can also train themselves to recognize when their thoughts are racing and to determine which thoughts they would prefer to focus on and which thoughts they would prefer not to entertain. Cannabis does not leave people powerless to control their thoughts and actions. Cannabis doesn't force people to think.

Everyone will navigate Cannabis much better if they can begin to recognize their individual patterns of hyperfocusing or having too many different thoughts running at the same time. Again, these "trains of thought" are something we all experience whether we consume Cannabis or not. These concepts may become much more noticeable or relatable after someone personally experiences increased neuron activity from psychoactive substances.

Hyperfocusing is interesting and is a fairly relatable phenomenon. New users might recall a "terrifying Cannabis moment" where they caught themselves staring at a random object or body part for an extended period of time. Anyone can find themselves fixating during times of "overthinking." People who regularly consume Cannabis can learn to recognize and control whether they want to be hyper-fixated on something or not. Experience might also teach someone that hyperfocusing can lead to new thoughts they might not have previously considered. Hyperfocusing on a single subject can introduce new ideas through thinking "deeper" into something. In other words, maybe it's not such a bad thing for someone to stare at their hand for five minutes and begin to hyper-fixate on who they really are and what they really want in life.

On the flip side, someone might recall a "terrifying Cannabis moment" where they couldn't "stay on subject" in their own thoughts. This could become overwhelming for someone who already has difficulty managing the wandering thoughts they don't prefer to have. Trauma and mental disorders may not be the easiest place to start, but with proper training and focus, anyone can learn and develop tips and tricks for how they prefer to manage their own thoughts.

Wandering thoughts are a "train of thought" that can take place while someone is trying to understand what someone else is saying. Someone might be trying to actively listen and become distracted by their own thoughts. Again, this might be a perfectly normal phenomenon for some people, but definitely not for everyone. Whichever the case, people can find themselves with racing thoughts during conversation. Like hyperfocusing, we can also learn to observe racing or unfocused thoughts, then learn to choose which thoughts to focus on.

Moments in creativity are great examples of how some of us might actually enjoy experiencing wandering thoughts while deciding what to do next and how to do it. It may not make everyone good at everything, but Cannabis can be an incredible influence for those who choose to pursue it. Thoughts in life are creative works of art in many ways. Thoughts are part of who we are as humans, and we should all have the freedom to manage our own minds with any substance of choice.

Reading comprehension is a great measure of someone's ability to focus and learn. If someone can learn to focus their thoughts while reading, then their "focus" will be improved. People can improve their focus both with and without Cannabis. Everyone who reads has experienced the phenomenon of reading something and completely forgetting to comprehend what they have just read. This is usually because they were too busy having other thoughts while they continued to mindlessly scan across words. Some people catch it quickly and only have to reread a couple words or lines, while others might read entire pages or paragraphs before realizing they need to go back and reread what they just read. With or without Cannabis, this is a perfectly normal part of reading comprehension. Practicing reading comprehension also helps build other conversational comprehension skills. Reading is an excellent tool for everyone to gauge, manage, and interact with their ability to focus during psychoactive activity.

Everyone has their own thoughts and actions to manage. Cannabis presents a choice of whether or not to consume it. Whether people consume Cannabis or not, everyone still has their own thoughts and actions to manage. Humans have the responsibility and universal right to manage their own thoughts and actions, and they should be provided the right to do so. Not allowing humans to consume Cannabis (or any other chosen substance) is the elimination of all free will of everyone who is affected.

Consideration 6

Ranking the Most Common Consumption Methods

Often when people think of consuming Cannabis, they think of smoking it. However, no one should smoke any burning substances—even if it's Cannabis. Many people do choose to regularly burn Cannabis, but that is not the only option for consumption. Smoking has become a major part of Cannabis culture, but smoking flower products is less beneficial when compared to other consumption methods.

On some level, any inhalation of any smoke is harmful. Some activists justify their smoking habit because they believe the benefits of Cannabis protect them. Even if this is true in a sense, smoking flower isn't the best option for anyone. That said, smoking flower is probably one of the loudest ways to "flex" the benefits of Cannabis on those who still continue to ignore the existence of Cannabis. Cannabis does provide benefits to people who smoke it, but just because someone consumes Cannabis, that doesn't make them invincible to developing dangerous habits that may not be ideal for lifelong use.

Activists will often share stories of personal justification as to why they choose to smoke. However, if an activist is truly serious in helping themselves and everyone else, then sharing actual consumption education is far more helpful than the whole "in your face" smoking approach. Some people do choose to smoke because they just don't care, just want to get stoned, or maybe just haven't realized that other consumption methods provide other advantages that smoking flower does not provide. Nobody should be criminalized for smoking, but people who do smoke should at least attempt to explore better forms of consumption so they can reduce smoking as much as possible.

Some smoking activists insist on smoking in public until the end of prohibition. The battle of activism has gotten us this far, and the need for it won't technically end until Cannabis prohibition is ended for everyone. Universal homegrowing is the only true way to ensure that the corruption of prohibition is completely eradicated. That said, both longtime activists and new consumers should avoid smoking flower by pursuing other consumption methods whenever possible. The pursuit of harm-reductive consumption is better for consumer safety and improving activism marketing in our local environments.

Activists who smoke flower are, in a way, playing into anti-Cannabis tactics. People who do not support Cannabis love the idea of "criminal" activists causing harm to themselves. People who choose to actively work against Cannabis may actually prefer consumers to smoke because they know it is more damaging to the reputation of Cannabis than marketing other forms of consumption, which are extremely difficult to argue against. Drug wars are real, and there are people and wealthy corporations who wish intentional harm against the Cannabis community. If the Cannabis community really wants to recruit everyone, then activists have got to improve their own consumption so the benefits can become clearer to everyone.

Activism was needed in the past to ensure that the medical benefits of Cannabis would never be ignored or erased from history completely. Today, medical Cannabis is regularly practiced, and education is available that shows just how useful Cannabis compounds can be. Now the Cannabis community needs to focus on how to continually improve methods of consumption and the products we choose to buy. Cannabis communities are empowered when their members become educated. Instead of teaching people that they have the right to smoke, now we can teach everyone how to be more harm-reductive in the selection of products and selected methods for consumption.

Consumption Method Rankings (from Best to Worst)

1. Nano-emulsion products
2. Edible foods, tinctures, and capsules

3. Skin applications (patches and salves)
4. Inhaling concentrates (dabs: rosin, resin, isolate, shatter, wax, oil, butter, crumble)
5. Flower vaporizing
6. Burning joints/pre-rolls
7. Burning flower in bongs and pipes
8. Burning "blunts" (Cannabis rolled in tobacco leaf) or "spliffs" (ground tobacco and Cannabis rolled with paper/leaf)

Pros and Cons for Each Method of Consumption

Nano-Emulsion Products

Pros
- No smoke or vapor entering the lungs
- Bypass initial gut and liver processing (increased bioavailability)
- Dispersed via bloodstream (faster onset than regular edibles)
- Premeasured doses save time in preparation
- No grinding, no heat, no device cleaning

Cons
- Usually the most expensive type of products
- Inaccurate formulations may not worth the higher price
- Contains non-Cannabis food ingredients (might not be beneficial)

Edible Foods, Tinctures, and Capsules:

Pros
- No smoke or vapor entering the lungs
- Premeasured doses save time in preparation
- No grinding, no heat, no device cleaning

Cons
- Contains non-Cannabis food ingredients (might not be beneficial)
- Processed by the gut and liver (decreased bioavailability)
- Dispersed via fats to which compounds are bound (slower onset)

Skin Applications (Patches and Salves):

Pros
- No smoke or vapor enters the lungs
- Premeasured doses save time in preparation
- No grinding, no heat, no device cleaning
- Can be made from a nano-emulsion formula (faster onset and bioavailability)
- Can target specific areas if inhalation or edible products are not effective in targeting specific areas that may benefit from more direct treatment(s)

Cons
- Contains non-Cannabis ingredients (might not be beneficial)
- Bioavailability VERY LOW if products are not nano-emulsified
- Dosing sizes may need to be increased due to lack of bioavailability
- High doses may be wasteful if bioavailability is too low
- Nano-emulsions usually the most expensive types of products

Vaporizing Concentrated Compounds:

Pros
- Less inhalation than flower to consume an equal amount of compounds
- Reduction in total carcinogens when compared to burning flower products
- Bypasses gut and liver processing (increased bioavailability)
- Transported by the bloodstream (faster onset)

Cons
- Vapor inhaled into the lungs
- Requires the purchase and utilization of a device designed for concentrates
- Requires device maintenance

Vaporizing Flower:

Pros
- Reduces carcinogens compared to burning flower
- Involves vapor inhalation BELOW 1000°F (538°C)
- Less inhalation than burning to consume an equal amount of compounds
- Bypasses initial gut and liver processing (increased bioavailability)
- Transported by the bloodstream (faster onset)

Cons
- Involves vapor inhalation into the lungs
- Requires the purchase and utilization of a vaporizer device
- Requires device maintenance
- Involves heated air inhalation
  - low temperatures allow cooler inhales, but require numerous inhalations
  - high temperatures require hotter inhalation, but allow fewer inhalations
  - cooling attachments are recommended because high temperatures do vaporize more quickly, but heated air best inhaled when cooled
  - lower temperatures may help preserve specific compounds, but the time spent to preserve certain compounds may not be worth the extra breaths of heated inhalation without proper cooling attachments

Burning Joints/Pre-Rolls:

Pros
- Cleaning of inhalation devices not required
- Rolling papers provide better flavor than smoking devices that taste like burned resin unless they are perfectly clean
- Bypasses initial gut and liver processing (increased bioavailability)

Cons

- Smoke reaches OVER 1000°F (538°C)
- Burning process creates additional carcinogens (decreased bioavailability)
- More inhalation than vaporizing to consume an equal amount of compounds
- More inhalation than concentrates to consume an equal amount of compounds
- Requires the additional purchase of rolling papers
- Requires the most preparation (and skill) compared to other consumption types
- Wastes many beneficial compounds when smoked and not vaporized, though some benefits still exist

Burning Flower in Bongs and Pipes:

Pros

- Grinding and loading a bowl faster than rolling a joint
- Bypasses initial gut and liver processing (increased bioavailability)
- Transported by the bloodstream (faster onset)

Cons

- Smoke reaches OVER 1000°F (538°C)
- Burning process creates additional carcinogens (decreased bioavailability)
- Requires constant cleaning to avoid tasting like burned resin
- Requires more inhalation than vaporizing to consume an equal amount of compounds
- Requires more inhalation than concentrates to consume an equal amount of compounds
- Requires the purchase and learning of a burning device
- Requires device maintenance
- Wastes many beneficial compounds when smoked and not vaporized, though some benefits still exist

Burning "Blunts" (Cannabis Rolled in Tobacco Leaf) or "Spliffs" (Ground Tobacco and Cannabis Rolled with Paper or Leaf):

Pros

- Tobacco provides nicotine to smokers, but tobacco is definitely never recommended for anybody's regular consumption. Vaping nicotine or tobacco contains lower temperatures and less carcinogens than burning tobacco leaves.
- Bypasses initial gut and liver processing (increased bioavailability)
- Transported by the bloodstream (faster onset)

Cons

- Smoke reaches OVER 1000°F (538°C)
- Burning process creates additional carcinogens (decreased bioavailability)
- Involves tobacco, which stopped being "doctor recommended" in 1964
- Requires more inhalation than vaporizing to consume an equal amount of compounds
- Requires more inhalation than concentrates to consume an equal amount of compounds
- Requires more inhalation than any other non-tobacco form of consumption
- Requires the additional purchase of tobacco
- Requires the most preparation (and skill) compared to other consumption types
- Wastes many beneficial compounds when smoked and not vaporized, though some benefits still exist

Now that you know the pros and cons of the various consumption methods, next we take a look at the different types of products available in the market today. It is important to choose products that align with your preferred methods of consumption.

Consideration 7

Common Types of Cannabis Products

Cannabis can be processed into many types of products. You should always be aware of product pricing and ensure you're buying enough specific compounds that are recommended for your specific treatments. Be aware of how many compounds are in a product and the price for each milligram. Be wary of companies that are selling "beautiful nuances," such as "premium packaging" or "premium effects" at a premium price. Premium "top-shelf" products may be superior compared to other products, but they are not the best solution if premium products keep you from affording your total recommended compounds.

Product Types

1. Flower
2. Concentrates
3. Edible Foods, Tinctures, Capsules
4. Skin Applications (Patches, Lotions, Bath Bombs, Salves)
5. Nano-Emulsion Products

Flower

Flower: the "nugs" of female Cannabis plants that are dried, trimmed, and cured for consumption

Product Consumption Methods

Flower can be vaporized, burned or processed into any other form of product.

Product Pricing

Distributor pricing may vary based on factors such as total compounds, exclusive brands, specialty strains, or seasonal pricing.

Flower can be machine-trimmed to reduce labor costs, but hand-trimming is typically key in creating "top-shelf" flower. Many manufacturers do insist that their flower products are hand-trimmed to avoid losing compounds that can be lost during machine-trimming and to help maximize profits by creating the best product possible.

Top-shelf products are generally more profitable to distributors, but bottom-shelf products may provide more compounds for the same price. Bottom-shelf products are not always "good deals," but they can be if they provide more compounds for a reduced price. You need to inspect pricing options carefully to determine which products will provide the most compounds for specific treatment recommendations. Product bioavailability must also be considered if two different types of products are being compared.

More Relevant Details

- Each Cannabis flower contains its own combination of compounds. Product labels should provide compound totals based on batch lab results. Labels should also include passing results from required contaminant testing.
- Flower is technically a "full-spectrum" product because compounds that are produced in flower are not lost during an extraction process.
- Flower can be processed into other product types. Raw flowers are less psychoactive until they are exposed to heat. This heating process is known as "decarboxylation" which converts THCA into THC (without the "A").

- Without complete "decarboxylation," THCA found in raw flower provides less psychoactive effects when eaten compared to a fully decarboxylated product.
- Regular edibles are usually less bioavailable than consuming flower.
- When eating raw flower, dried and cured flower will provide slightly more psychoactive effects than freshly picked flower because small amounts of THCA are converted into THC through minor decarboxylation that can take place during the drying and curing processes.
- THCA cannot efficiently bind to CB1 & CB2 receptors in the body that would otherwise contribute to psychoactive effects. This is why decarboxylation is such a critical part of compound consumption.
- It may be cost-effective to make certain products from flower rather than buying other premade products. This is only true if the "decarboxylation" processes are properly executed, however. Affordable edibles may or may not be as affordable compared to flower, but it's important not to waste flower purchases due to improper decarboxylation processing.
- Consuming flower involves more inhalation of total plant material than inhaling an equivalent amount of concentrated compounds. This may not seem to matter when it comes to daily consumption, but this detail can make a HUGE difference in reducing total inhalations during long-term consumption strategies.

Concentrates

Concentrates: produced by collecting and/or manipulating compounds from Cannabis using various extraction, separation, and/or conversion methods

Product Consumption Methods
Concentrates can be vaporized, burned, or processed into any other product except flower.

Product Pricing

Distributor pricing may vary based on total compounds, exclusive brands, specialty strains, or seasonal pricing.

Concentrates can be farmed and extracted using large-scale processes to reduce labor costs, but competitive top-shelf products can be difficult to achieve on a large scale. Manufacturers who are not able to farm and extract on a large scale may find themselves struggling to offer prices that are competitive with professional large-scale production. When purchasing Cannabis, you should always shop around to find the best quality products with the best pricing available.

Top-shelf products are generally more profitable to distributors, but bottom-shelf products may provide more compounds for the same price. Bottom-shelf products are not always "good deals," but they can be if they provide more compounds for a reduced price. It's important to inspect pricing options carefully to determine which products will provide the most compounds for specific treatment recommendations. Product bioavailability must also be considered when comparing two different types of products.

More Relevant Details

- Product labels should provide compound totals based on batch lab results. Labels should also include passing results for contaminant testing. This is especially important for concentrates that use chemicals that are not intended for end-product consumption.
- Concentrate products require quality flower, specific extraction equipment, flower compounds, and precise processing in order to achieve top-shelf quality.
- Some concentrates only contain one type of compound, or they might contain a collection of a few different compounds. In general, top-shelf concentrates intend to preserve every compound possible produced by a Cannabis plant.
- **Certain extraction methods include the use of harsh chemicals that require full removal of chemicals prior to consumption. Only consume chemically extracted concentrates if testing**

results have proven that there are no harsh chemicals leftover from the extraction process.

- Another way to avoid consuming leftover chemicals is to select products that are extracted without the use of harsh chemicals. Even still, solventless concentrates (made without any chemicals) must pass contaminant testing prior to consumption.

- Disposable "vape cartridges" reduce preparation and cleanup.

- Dabbing devices without preset options should be used with a temperature reading device. Devices with presets are designed to avoid accidental high-temperature dabbing consumption.

- Optimal device temperatures will vary depending on the type of concentrate and the amount of compounds someone is needing to consume for their recommended treatments.

- Low temperatures help preserve compounds that are destroyed at high temperatures, but they may not fully vaporize other compounds. Concentrates may be reheated if they are not fully vaporized the first time they are heated.

- Temperatures that are too hot will lower bioavailability of compounds if they are burned to smoke rather than vaporized. Check product labels to determine which temperatures are best to avoid wasting certain compounds that are recommended for treatments.

- Super-heated inhalations of burned smoke material should always be avoided. Always use sufficient cooling attachments to remove as much excess heat as possible.

- Some people claim they prefer flower because of its "full-spectrum" effects. However, not all concentrates are created equal. There are a variety of extraction techniques designed to preserve the exact same spectrum of compounds that are found in the flower from which they are extracted.

Many prefer flower for personal habit reasons; flower is certainly enjoyable to many people. However, flower does not provide any special compounds that wouldn't also be found in a full-spectrum concentrate.

Inhaling flower requires more plant material to be inhaled into the lungs than inhaling concentrated compounds. Unlike flower, concentrates can be filtered to eliminate certain compounds that may not be recommended for inhalation treatments. Flower only contains the compounds produced by the plant from which they are harvested. Concentrates can contain any spectrum of different compounds because extractions can come from more than one plant.

In a world full of untested extraction products, the flower-only logic can make a lot of sense. Untested flower can still contain contaminants that would never pass actual testing, but untested extracts could contain leftover processing chemicals that could make them more dangerous if potentially harmful chemicals are used in the extraction process. Concentrates should definitely be avoided if you aren't sure which extraction chemicals were used or if products have not passed contamination testing.

Medical experts don't sell or recommend untested concentrates to anyone. Medical distributors are typically only allowed to sell tested concentrates that can be recommended as a better alternative to flower.

Edible Foods, Tinctures, Capsules

Edible Foods, Tinctures, Capsules: decarboxylated and mixed with oil, alcohol, or even water if compounds are properly nano-emulsified.

Product Consumption Methods
Under the tongue, chewable, or single-swallow

Product Pricing
Distributor pricing may vary based on total compounds, exclusive brands, specialty strains, or seasonal pricing.

Edibles can be some of the cheapest products available or they can be some of the most expensive. Edible products are usually more expensive per 1mg/THC when compared to buying flower or concentrate products. If prices do seem relatively close, then you can also consider the bioavailability of the compared products.

Low-quality edibles can lack bioavailability. Improper decarboxylation makes for reduced bioavailability. Edible products lack bioavailability unless compounds are nano-emulsified. Nano-sized edibles actually have the best bioavailability compared to any other type of product, but most edible products are not nano-emulsified. Improper compound sizing can result in similar bioavailability as regular edibles if compounds are too large. Compounds that are too small also have the potential to be less bioavailable. Edibles that are nano-sized are only the most bioavailable type of products if the compounds have been sized properly.

Top-shelf products are generally more profitable to distributors, but bottom-shelf products may provide more compounds for the same price. Bottom-shelf products are not always "good deals," but they can be if they provide more compounds for a reduced price. You may need to inspect pricing options carefully to determine which products will provide you with the most compounds for your specific treatment recommendations. Product bioavailability must also be considered when comparing two different types of products.

More Relevant Details

- Onset times are determined by size of dose, personal tolerance, daily metabolism/diet/exercise, and accuracy of the decarboxylation process. Some packaging may indicate estimated onset times, but be aware that everyone will have their own variable results.

- Edible products contain their own combination of compounds. Product labels should provide total compounds based on lab results. Labels should also include passing results from contaminant testing.

- Edible products are created by infusing either flower or concentrate with other edible ingredients.

- There is the potential of containing other ingredients that some may or may not want to consume regularly or during treatments. Examples of this include artificial ingredients, sweeteners, or other foods people may be better off avoiding.

- Products may contain compound mixtures such as 50mgTHC, 50mgCBD, and 50mgCBG. Mixed compound products typically contain compounds that have been extracted from multiple species of Cannabis. The main thing to ensure with this type of mixed products is to avoid paying high THC prices for non-THC compounds that can be purchased much more inexpensively.
- Products can be nano-sized for faster onset times and better bioavailability, but nano-emulsified products are generally more expensive per milligram.
- Edible concentrates should not be vaporized or smoked. It isn't recommended to inhale ingredients that are not intended for inhalation. Don't vaporize concentrated products that contain food ingredients not intended for inhalation.

Skin Applications (Patches, Lotions, Bath Bombs, Salves)

Skin Applications (Patches, Lotions, Bath Bombs, Salves): can be used to pinpoint specific pains/ailments but not be absorbed into the skin unless properly nano-emulsified

Product Consumption Methods
Applied to skin as directed by product labels

Product Pricing
Distributor pricing may vary based on total compounds, exclusive brands, specialty strains, or seasonal pricing.

If skin application products are not nano-sized or completely absorbed into the skin, then Cannabis compounds are pretty much just on the label for show. Skin products may be helpful or beneficial due to certain ingredients, but Cannabis compounds will have pretty much non-existent bioavailability unless they are nano-emulsified. Skin products can be effective for treatments, but bioavailability is extremely low if products are not formulated for their intended application method.

Top-shelf products are generally more profitable to distributors, but bottom-shelf products may provide more compounds for the same price. Bottom-shelf products are not always "good deals," but they can be if they provide more compounds for a reduced price. Inspect pricing options carefully to determine which products provide the most compounds for specific treatment recommendations. Product bioavailability must also be considered when comparing two different types of products.

More Relevant Details
- Products can be used to target specific areas if inhalation or edible applications are not effective in targeting a specific area or condition in need of treatments.
- Commonly more expensive per 1mg/THC compared to buying any other products due to the lack of bioavailability. The only exceptions to this are nano-emulsified skin applications, which are also usually pretty expensive.

Nano-Emulsion Products

Nano-emulsion products are compounds that are "emulsified" until compound molecules are whipped into measured nano-particle sizes that are not too big or too small. Properly sized formulations are water soluble and can be used to create a variety of fast-onset products. They are also the most bioavailable method of consuming Cannabis compounds.

Product Consumption Methods
Under the tongue, chewable, single-swallow, or applied to skin as directed by product labels

Product Pricing
Distributor pricing may vary based on total compounds, exclusive brands, specialty strains, or current season prices on existing inventory.

Nano-emulsions are usually pretty expensive. They do have the best bioavailability, but they require specific formulations for that to be true. These formulations require tools to measure nano-particle sizes, equipment to create nano-sized compounds, and people who know how to make all of those things happen successfully. That said, there are distributors who make affordable nano-emulsion products because they know this is the best option for patients who need or prefer high bioavailability of the compounds they consume.

Top-shelf products are generally more profitable to distributors, but bottom-shelf products may provide more compounds for the same price. Bottom-shelf products are not always "good deals," but they can be if they provide more compounds for a reduced price. Inspect pricing options carefully to determine which products will provide the most compounds for specific treatment recommendations. Product bioavailability must also be considered when comparing two different types of products.

More Relevant Details

- Nano-sized compounds have a fast onset and the best bioavailability compared to any other form of consumption.
- Labels usually say "fast-acting," or they might provide estimated onset times.
- Regular (non-nano) high-dose edible cannabinoids must be processed by the liver because compounds are attached to fats that the body is only able to distribute after the compound-rich fats have been processed.

Nano-emulsified products are dispersed throughout the body without the need of liver processing because nano-sized compounds are water-soluble. The body may be able to utilize nano-sized compounds more thoroughly throughout the body.

Not bypassing the liver could become problematic in the long run or maybe even in the short term for certain people with existing liver conditions. That said, the liver processing of various compounds could also benefit people with liver conditions in recommended quantities. People with existing liver conditions could consider this possibility. They should consult medical professionals on what is best for their specific situation and current state of their conditions.

Consideration 8

Examples for Budgeting High/Low Dosages and Not Paying THC Prices for Legal Compounds

Some people prefer small or occasional dosings, while others might require dosages that are either more frequent or much larger. Where homegrowing isn't allowed, consumers will need to purchase products sold by locally available distributors.

If a person cannot consistently afford their recommended compounds and lifelong use is expected, they actually may need or want to consider relocating somewhere where they are able to safely afford their recommended dosages. Homegrowing is by far the most affordable option of accessing Cannabis, especially if high-dose recommendations are to be expected.

Without insurance coverage, most people are left facing the major expense of Cannabis products on their own. People who cannot afford Cannabis are likely to become customers of other non-Cannabis alternatives. Other commonly consumed substances have already been shown to cause more death and more harmful effects than Cannabis, year after year.

Recreational and medical distributors are not affordable options for people who can only afford Cannabis with insurance coverage. Most people don't realize that Cannabis is only expensive because they aren't allowed to homegrow. In places where Cannabis can be legally homegrown, people are able to find gardeners, farmers, family, or friends who are happy to help them produce their own Cannabis compounds.

People don't always calculate how much money they spend on Cannabis. Cannabis is often viewed as "well worth the cost" by those who regularly make the decision to buy it. However, there are plenty of people out there who struggle financially and don't understand how financially damaging overpriced products can become over time. It's important for everyone to understand the difference between common distributor pricing and homegrowing.

The Financial Impacts of People Who Consume Low-Doses versus High-Doses of Cannabis

Let's look at two examples of Cannabis consumers. Patient One only consumes Cannabis at night to help with sleep. Patient Two deals with 24/7 chronic pain and consumes Cannabis periodically throughout their day. Without Cannabis, Patient One sleeps terribly, and Patient Two experiences constant pain. Both patients prefer Cannabis because other sleeping pills and pain pills include side effects that they want to avoid.

Getting to Know Patient One

Patient One consumes 50mg/THC an hour or two before bed. THC helps them relax before and during sleep. THC also benefits other systems in their body. If Patient One is consuming 20%THC flower, then they would only be consuming ¼/g. In other words, it takes them four days to consume a single 1g/joint.

50MG/THC can be overwhelming for some people, especially for those who are new to Cannabis. Others, such as Patient Two, might barely notice the effects of 50mg/THC if they are used to consuming 500mg/THC/Day for their needs.

At 50mg/THC/Day, Patient One probably won't be very successful in treating severe chronic pain. However, small amounts of THC could help someone in pain by helping them reduce or even eventually replace their pain pills with Cannabis. Patients should consult their medical professionals to explore reducing or replacing their pain pills with Cannabis.

People who require management of significant pain could easily require more than 2.5g of 20%THC/Flower throughout their day. Again, people can benefit from 50mg/THC, but for managing significant pain, 50mg/THC will likely fall short of what should be recommended.

Getting to Know Patient Two

Patient Two consumes THC periodically all day long. THC helps Patient Two manage excessive pain. THC also benefits other systems in Patient Two's body. Patients who live in constant pain may prefer to consume as much Cannabis as they can physically tolerate or as much as they can afford—perhaps a set amount such as 2.5g/20%THC/Flower/Day (500MG/THC) for budgeting purposes.

If you have chronic pain, you should start with a low dose and go slow while exploring your tolerance to Cannabis compounds. This is especially true if recommendations are expected to be large or frequent. Keep in mind that large or frequent doses might not always be the ideal solution, however.

For comparison, Patient One, who benefits from sleep assistance, consumes less Cannabis in an entire week (350mg/THC/week) than Patient Two, who benefits from pain management by consuming 500mg/THC in a single day. If you are new to Cannabis, you may want or even need to work with a Cannabis expert. Cannabis experts can help you gradually explore higher doses of Cannabis as required.

Patient One Budgeting for 50mg/THC/Day in Medical and Recreational Markets

Patient One might spend between $0.03 and $0.15+ for 1mg of THC depending on the distributors they choose and the products they buy.

This common price ranges leaves Patient One to finance the following potential budget estimates:

50mg/THC/day= $1.50-$7.50+

350mg/THC/week= $10.50-$52.50+

1,400mg/THC/month= $42-$210+

16,800mg/THC/year= $504-$2,520+

*REMINDER: 50mg/day may be sufficient for some people, overwhelming for others, but for some people, 50mg/day might fall very short of what they might actually need or prefer.

Patient Two Budgeting for 500mg/THC/Day in Medical and Recreational Markets

Patient Two might spend between $0.03 and $0.15+ for 1mg of THC depending on the distributors they choose and the products they buy. This common price range means that Patient Two must finance the following potential budget estimates:

500mg/THC/day= $15-$75+

3500mg/THC/week= $105-$525+

14,000mg/THC/month= $420-$2100+

168,000mg/THC/year= $5,040-$25,200+

*REMINDER: Some people may require or would prefer to consume far more than just 500mg/THC/day. Doses of that size make medical and recreational Cannabis impossible for most people to afford without homegrowing options. Even if they can afford high doses, they might not be willing to pay such a high price for something that could be easily homegrown. If homegrowing is legalized, people would be able to grow their own Cannabis for a FRACTION of the cost because they don't have to help finance the overhead costs of local distributors such as employee labor, property rent, plant cultivation, and product manufacturing. This is especially true for people who already have gardens that already produce other plants. Learning to grow Cannabis is possible with the help and assistance of other experienced growers, garden supply stores, farmers, or experienced gardeners.

For Educational Purposes

One single Cannabis plant can produce between 1/oz and over 10 pounds of flower. Garden supply stores are able to provide full education on budgeting and growing your very own Cannabis. Homegrowing remains ILLEGAL for those who live in communities where people lack education about the many benefits of Cannabis.

Don't Pay THC Prices for Legal Compounds That Can Be Purchased Online

Compounds that are federally legal are typically more affordable at locations where THC is not sold. Certain THC distributors may carry other compounds at a reduced price, but most of the time, people will find that other compounds are typically much cheaper online or in other retail stores. Other compounds are more affordable because they are able to be legally farmed on a much larger scale. The largest legal THC grow in the nation is just over two hundred acres, while non-THC compounds are legally farmed on hundreds and even thousands of acres.

For instance, some states might only allow THC licenses to farm up to a certain amount of land or they may not allow farmers to grow THC at all. Farmers who are allowed to grow five acres of THC may be allowed to grow thousands of acres of CBD.

It may be beneficial to consume other compounds alongside THC, but other compounds are usually much cheaper when purchased from non-THC distributors. The key is to shop around, research product reviews, look at lab results for total compounds, make sure no contaminants were found, calculate the price per milligram, and don't pay an extra-high price just for more expensive packaging.

There are companies that offer high-quality compounds for less than $.05/per mg. There are many farms throughout the country who are happy to sell non-THC orders online, over the phone, or in person.

We all should avoid paying THC prices for other recommended compounds by price shopping online or at local grocery stores and gas stations. Buying directly from a farm will usually beat out other available pricing, but all products do require lab testing prior to any legal sale. Those who can reduce their price per/1mg of compound will increase the total amount of compounds they can afford for their consumption in medical or recreational markets.

Example Rankings for Selecting THC Products

Based on 5 grams of flower that all contain a concentration of 20% total compounds:

1. $50: 20%THC = 1000mgTHC
2. $50: 15%THC/5%CBD = 750mgTHC/250mgCBD
3. $50: 10%THC/10%CBD = 500mgTHC/500mgCBD
4. $50: 5%THC/10%CBD/5%CBG= 250mgTHC/500mgCBD/ 250mgCBG

In this example, all four options are $50 each and priced at $0.05 for every 1 mg of compound. Option 1 is the best option because THC is the most expensive compound on the market. Option 4 contains the least amount of THC and still ranks last even though it is the only option with THC, CBD, and CBG. If a distributor is selling other compounds for the same price as THC, it would be best to purchase non-THC compounds from other distributors.

Homegrowing different compounds is possible wherever it is legal to do so. Homegrowing will always be the most affordable access to Cannabis for most of us.

Consideration 9

The Importance of Increasing Tolerance for THC

When it comes to teaching people about "THC tolerance," I often find myself cringing on the inside. Some individuals say that "THC tolerance" is something that happens to people who decide that their recommended dosages are "no longer effective" because their "tolerance for THC" has made their size of dosage less effective than before.

Describing tolerance in this way only makes sense if someone isn't able to afford enough compounds for their own needs. If someone is unable to afford increased dosages because their tolerance becomes "too high," then the problem is not their tolerance. Instead of suggesting increased dosages, this method suggests that consumers in treatment should take a "tolerance-break" so they won't have to increase their dosages if they are unable to afford increased dosages.

My Approach to THC Tolerance

My approach to "THC tolerance" is much different than what others often describe. I teach that if we are not prepared or capable of increasing our thresholds for THC, we may eventually find ourselves in a place where larger doses are needed, and we will want to be in a position to enjoy those larger dosages as much as possible.

I believe that THC tolerance is how much THC someone can consume before feeling overwhelmed. No matter how it's consumed, too much THC can make someone physically sick or can result in experiencing thoughts that may be personally challenging or seem inescapable. A person's tolerance for THC can vary from day to day, week to week, or even year to year. THC tolerance is affected by factors such as regularity of use, personal beliefs, daily metabolism, daily mood, and daily living environments.

It is possible for consumers to feel overwhelmed by a certain THC dose recommendation because other benefits may be needed or desirable. If THC is difficult or overwhelming for someone, that person may need to put in some effort to increase their tolerance for THC. Effort can be personally managed, but some may require additional professional assistance from medical professionals or other available support systems. Building tolerance for THC means learning to enjoy and prefer larger doses of THC without getting physically sick or mentally overwhelmed. It's not just being able to tolerate Cannabis, but also enjoying the pursuit of its recommended benefits as much as humanly possible.

THC is probably the only Cannabis compound most of us will encounter "tolerance issues" with. Some consumers might be overwhelmed with just 10-50mg/THC. Meanwhile, those same people might barely notice if they consumed 100mg-1000mg of other non-psychoactive compounds such as CBG, CBN, or CBD. There are also people who get overwhelmed with 10-50mg/THC, but who are recommended to consume 100-1000+mg/THC/Day based on their specific needs. Someone might need to increase their personal tolerance if the recommended doses are more than they are able to tolerate.

Without learning to enjoy THC, people may completely give up THC and gravitate again to other consumable substances that might contribute less beneficial effects, more pain, declining health, or other worsened life outcomes. If someone is having trouble getting comfortable with THC, they might want to consider searching for educated Cannabis experts or educated Cannabis communities that are capable of supporting Cannabis consumers in building and understanding their personal tolerance and preferences for the psychoactive effects of THC.

Learning to overcome tolerance for recommended dosages may be a challenging process if you are consuming compounds without the support of educational resources. Learning to prefer THC is very helpful in the long run. The process of enjoying preferences is far less challenging once tolerance issues are overcome.

Too much THC can lead to what is known as a "non-lethal overdose." This is just another way of saying that someone might be overwhelmed, but they won't die. Anyone who experiences a non-lethal THC overdose is encouraged to sleep, meditate, pray, eat, hydrate, and try to be as calm as they can. When someone is overwhelmed, it's important to realize that Cannabis is not the cause of uncomfortable or uncontrollable thoughts.

Overwhelming experiences may involve either passing thoughts or ongoing patterns of thought that may seem uncontrollable or inescapable. The effects of Cannabis cannot be blamed for anyone's failure to learn or develop their tolerance for the psychoactive effects of THC. The issue isn't Cannabis. The issues belong to the person with tolerance issues. Cannabis will do what it does for the body whether someone else prefers the psychoactivity of THC or not.

Cannabis does not dictate what anyone's thoughts will be, but it can affect the speed and number of thoughts that seem to be observed or communicated by consumers of THC. Before moving forward with larger doses, doses should be kept small until a person is able to get familiar and be comfortable with psychoactive activity. That said, there may be situations where high doses are immediately called for—for instance, in cases where pain is severe and ongoing. It's very useful to develop tolerance for large doses before any severe pain is ever present. However, without educational preparation, large doses of THC may be difficult to tolerate.

Each individual must determine whether they prefer smaller doses to manage pain or if larger doses are required. The best advice I can give is to recognize that Cannabis isn't going to cause lethal overdose, even though it may be overwhelming. Tolerance *can* be learned and developed rather quickly with proper navigation. And of course, if someone chooses to give up on Cannabis, other non-Cannabis alternatives can be prescribed by medical professionals.

People in serious pain typically won't have much choice but to consume large amounts of THC in order to effectively manage their pain, whether they prefer it or not. If they can't learn to tolerate Cannabis, they may decide to leverage other effective alternatives that may or may not come with long lists of "side effects."

Other alternatives to Cannabis may be statistically more harmful or dangerous for consumption. Ask your medical professionals what other options they might recommend for your specific treatments and tolerance situation. Hopefully, those medical professionals will be capable and willing to recommend Cannabis, especially if other alternatives are known and expected to cause additional complications in your life.

Providing personalized Cannabis recommendations to their patients may be difficult or impossible for medical professionals who are not actual experts in Cannabis. You may need to seek medical professionals who specifically recommend Cannabis to people on a regular basis in order to receive accurate recommendations and guidance. Extra bonus if you are able to find medical professionals who specialize in your specific health issues and regularly recommend Cannabis using appropriate small, medium, large or mega-sized dosages based on recommended treatments and personal preferences.

After visiting medical experts and Cannabis experts, do some additional research. Always fact-check any advice you receive because you want to make sure that the received recommendations match the recommendations provided by other Cannabis experts. You can only develop our daily preferences through personal experience and deciding for yourself. You can benefit when consuming small doses of THC, but large and frequent THC dosing recommendations are often required for specific treatments.

If someone is recommended to consume large and frequent dosings, affordability should not hold them back from doing so. Cost often limits recommended consumption, but if high doses are recommended, then homegrowing may be the only route to affording the dosages that are recommended for consumption. If prices are too high, then we need to discover ways to access Cannabis as safely and affordably as possible. If homegrowing isn't legal, it may not be safe for you to pursue Cannabis. If it isn't legal, hopefully laws will be created so Cannabis can become less financially problematic to those who are recommended to consume unaffordable dosages of Cannabis compounds.

We should consume as much Cannabis as we prefer or need, but we should also realize that recommended dosages vary depending on the types of products and methods of consumption used over periods of time. Protecting the finances of consumers is also EXTREMELY important because saving people money is part of service to others. If someone cannot afford dosages in their area and if they are not allowed to homegrow, then they may choose to relocate so they can rightfully and safely access the recommended dosages for their treatment.

We should seek Cannabis experts who can help guide us in maintaining elevated THC levels in the body as comfortably and enjoyable as possible. Many medical professionals have no idea how to properly recommend Cannabis to their patients. Many have never taken Cannabis themselves and don't understand how to properly prepare people for long-term or even short-term Cannabis consumption.

Most medical professionals today have never considered many of the important topics that this book describes. This is often because it doesn't make much sense for medical professionals to pursue something that might cause them to lose high-priced medical degrees and practices. Cannabis should have never left the "medical wheelhouse," but since it did, many medical professionals have been happy to maintain the narrative that Cannabis does not belong. Cannabis should be the base of every "medical wheelhouse," like water, like exercise, like therapy, and especially like forms of daily pain management. Politicians and religious agendas are to blame, not medical professionals. Medical professionals MUST recognize the reality that Cannabis is beneficial to everyone, and politicians and religious leaders should help establish and protect the consumption and homegrowing of Cannabis for everyone. Cannabis is good for everyone.

That said, medical professionals have the right to their opinion, and they can still be appreciated for choosing to help people to the best of their knowledge and ability. This book is intended to make things clear as to why everyone should definitely be recommending Cannabis to every person who drinks, inhales smoke, or consumes any other less beneficial substance than Cannabis. This book is not intended to make anyone look bad, but rather to shed light on the systemic misinformation that still exists today.

Understanding the prices of Cannabis is important for people who only have medical insurance that covers non-Cannabis pharmaceutical medications. It takes a real Cannabis expert to guide people in how to provide Cannabis for themselves most affordably or how to access a community who can help Cannabis be more affordable in their local area.

Every treatment has its place in the medical field, and medical professionals are responsible for providing everyone with the best recommendations possible. Cannabis might not treat every condition, but it should be extremely rare to tell anyone that they should not consume Cannabis compounds. Medical professionals cannot be expected to know everything. Their opinions should be considered when ultimately determining what will or will not be consumed during any recommendation for any medical condition.

Most medical professionals won't know how they can best recommend Cannabis compounds unless they do additional research outside their previous understandings of Cannabis. That said, this book hopes to inspire medical professionals to further their Cannabis education and to expand upon the many considerations found in this book. If medical professionals do not get a real education in Cannabis, then they won't be prepared to provide Cannabis recommendations for their patients.

Medical professionals who are educated in Cannabis should be able to help new consumers navigate high or low dosings for their recommended treatments. They should also be able to help them plan to be as "harm-reductive" in their consumptions as possible. This can be a difficult thing to explain without firsthand experience, but ongoing long-term (month-to-month or year-to-year) and short-term (day-to-day) strategies can be developed. Strategies must be based on the specific needs and preferences of individuals.

Genuine experts in Cannabis should be able to suggest strategic plans for increasing someone's total THC/mg/day most comfortably if existing tolerance levels are low. Recommendations should include as many details as possible, such as:

- How many and which specific compounds are best for treating specific conditions
- Where to buy products and how homegrowing can significantly reduce costs
- How to start with small tolerable doses and increase slowly or quickly as needed
- Best time of day for someone to consume specific compounds
- Specific methods that should be used for various compound consumptions
- How to utilize a variety of Cannabis compounds such as CBD, CBG, terpenes, and other natural Cannabis oils/compounds so they may pursue a variety of benefits or to encourage improvements or relief for a specific condition.
- Recommendations for therapy sessions for those who may benefit from resolving or preparing to experience a potential increase of personally troubling thoughts

Some people who experience chronic pain might prefer just 10mg-50mg/THC at night to aid in sleep because they don't like taking more than that; mission accomplished. On the other hand, there are people with chronic pain or other diseases where the recommended strategy may be to flood the body with as much THC as possible. Recommendations for 1,000mg+/THC/day are possible. Some people might even aim to consume as much THC as physically tolerable in order to treat "hard to reach" places in the body or to reach as much of the body as physically possible. Some individuals may need to maintain high and frequent dosings for the rest of their life.

Consideration 10

Comparing Inhalation Products and Determining the Quality and Safety of Cannabis Products

The Difference Between Inhaling THC Flower and Inhaling Concentrated THC Products

The consumption rankings in Consideration 6 provided further detail as to why inhaling flower is not the best option for consumption. Basically, consuming flower involves inhalation of plant material that is removed when concentrated Cannabis products are made. Concentrated products are superior to less concentrated products because less total material can be consumed to receive an equal amount of compounds. Many claim to prefer flower for its flavor or effects, but those people should be aware of the time, cost savings, refined flavors and self-preservation that comes when flower inhalation is either replaced or reduced by consuming higher concentrated products instead.

For this comparison, let's revisit Patient One and Patient Two from Consideration 8. The consumption levels of these two patients will show just how big of a difference there is when comparing the inhalation of flower and concentrated products. Patient One consumes 50mg/THC/Day to help them get to sleep and Patient Two consumes 500mg/THC/Day for 24/7 management of severe chronic pain. Notice that both patients are able to inhale far less material into their lungs when concentrated products are consumed instead of flower. In fact, the product examples below allow both patients to inhale four times less material into their lungs if they choose to consume the 80% concentrated THC product instead of a 20% THC flower.

No one should be forced into inferior consumption methods due to affordability. Flower products may seem less expensive, but concentrated products are clearly better solutions for consumers when considering the potential or likelihood of long-term consumptions of THC.

The key takeaway from this consideration is that inhaling flower is not as beneficial when compared to inhaling concentrated products that contain an equal amount of THC.

Patient One consumes 50mg/THC/Day before sleep:

Total MG:	20%THC/Flower:		80%THC/Concentrate:
50mg/day	0.25g/Flower	OR	0.0625g/Concentrate
350mg/week	1.75g/Flower	OR	0.4375g/Concentrate
1,400mg/month	7g/Flower	OR	1.75g/Concentrate
16,800mg/year	84g/Flower	OR	21g/Concentrate

NOTICE: Inhaling 84g/20%THC/Flower/year would involve four times as much inhalation as inhaling just 21g/80%THC/Concentrate/year.

Patient Two consumes 500mg/THC/Day for 24/7 chronic pain management:

Total MG:	20%THC/Flower:		80%THC/Concentrate:
500mg/day	2.5g/Flower	OR	0.625g/Concentrate
3500mg/week	17.5g/Flower	OR	4.375g/Concentrate
14000mg/month	70g/Flower	OR	17.5g/Concentrate
168,000mg/year	840g/Flower	OR	210/g/Concentrate

NOTICE: Inhaling 840g/20%THC/Flower/year would involve four times as much inhalation as inhaling just 210g/80%THC/Concentrate/year.

Determining the Quality and Safety of Cannabis Products

Many people are not allowed to consume Cannabis for treatment, either because they don't have legal distributors in their area or they can't afford their recommended dosages in their local medical or recreational markets. This drives some people into buying criminalized Cannabis where lab testing is unregulated and unwanted contaminants are possible.

We all have the following options for accessing Cannabis:

- Find a grower
- Find a distributor
- Hire a grower
- Visit a hydroponic/garden store for growing supplies and/or advice so we can homegrow it ourselves

Homegrowing allows us all to ensure that our products are not contaminated with harmful chemicals or pesticides. Just because a product is legally produced doesn't mean the product hasn't been produced with "approved" chemicals and/or pesticides.

Regardless of where a product comes from, we should always consider the following while inspecting products for quality:

1. Untested products can be dangerous or misleading. Good lab results will provide potency of various compounds and if any contaminants are present. Lab testing is the only way to accurately determine an unknown product's potency and cleanliness.
2. If anyone plans to consume untested products, then they may be at risk of consuming contaminants, or they might end up with different compounds than expected. Cannabis can absorb heavy metals and other contaminants via water, soil, or added nutrients. Even some of the best growers can fail testing due to unexpected contaminants. Contaminants can come from rainwater, local

water, poor quality soil, or contaminated nutrients. Without end-product testing, potential contaminants and potency cannot be known.

3. How does it smell? Cannabis is well known for its floral, gasoline, fruity, sour, and skunky aromas. Smells can come from specific terpenes, or they can come from contaminants such as mold. If it smells like mold, we should visually inspect it for either white mold or dark "bud rot," which can be found by breaking open contaminated nugs. If flower smells like hay, the strain could be lacking in terpenes. Hay smells can also be a sign that flower material was either not dried slowly enough or it has not had enough time to properly develop its fragrance. Hay smells in recently harvested material may be remedied by proper drying and storage. This drying and storage process is critical and is known as the curing process.

4. How does it look? Some Cannabis flowers might seem more fluffy, dense, seedy, or frosty than others. Know what to look for and what it might mean.

   - None of us want to consume white mold, loose hair, or other visible contaminants. Some flower products can have more potential for mold because moisture can become trapped inside the core of the product. Whenever possible, buyers should ask to inspect untested flower products by breaking up a couple larger nugs to ensure there isn't any visible mold inside the product.

   - Growing conditions and genetics are both factors that affect the density, size, and shape of raw flower products. Flowers might look like scrambled fluffy clouds, or they may appear as dense solid nuggets. These flower structures could mean a few things. Scrambled or fluffy cloud-like nugs may have been grown in too much heat, too much light, not enough CO_2, or not enough water. Dense solid buds are generally a sign of better growing conditions. The logic in comparing the two would be to assume that denser flower is a sign of better end product. That said, denser flower does not mean there will be more beneficial compounds. Some genetics are simply fluffier than others. Comparing the structure can be helpful when trying to make specific comparisons, except most of the time gauging the appearance of "frost" is generally more relevant than comparing structure.

- The structure of flower is one thing; how a nug frosts and shines is another. Those sticky-shiny sparkles are called *trichomes*, and they store various compounds produced by the plant. The more trichomes, the more beneficial compounds. If products seem equally "shiny," then it may be helpful to do some additional research. If strain names are known, research can provide information on which cannabinoids are likely to be found within the shiny trichomes of those strains. This is helpful because if there is a strain that has been likely to produce higher amounts of THC, then the trichomes that are present will also be more likely to contain higher concentrations of THC.

- Seeded flowers are produced by female plants that were either pollinated by males or overly stressed during their growing process. Males produce seeds and do not produce the same compound-bearing "nugs" as females. Nugs can contain many seeds; these are not recommended for inhalation. In addition, seeds can be very tedious to remove. Cannabis seeds are one of the best sources of plant protein, but they rarely contain as many compounds as flowers that don't contain any seeds.

  - Growing seeds can take months of work, and growing random seeds is not recommended. If a seed doesn't contain strong feminized genetics, growers are at risk of only growing more seeds instead of compound-rich flower material that is free from undesired seeds. It is best to either use clones from a female mother plant that is known to produce seedless flower or source feminized seeds from a reputable seed distributor or Cannabis breeder. Seeds can be shipped and sold worldwide because THC is prohibited but seeds are not. And sometimes, clones are legal too.

5. Consumption inspection: If someone pays THC prices, they should receive THC. Were the effects desirable? Does the buyer feel the price was worth the value? Are they able to afford enough product to consume their recommended dosages until they are able to buy more? Can the buyer rely on the same distributor if they run out sooner than expected? These are the questions we must answer for ourselves before returning to the same distributor.

Consideration 11

Cannabis Preparation Checklist and Troubleshooting Tips

The following checklist and troubleshooting tips are designed to provide you with quick ideas that are good to keep in mind while in pursuit of Cannabis. Whether you have been consuming Cannabis for decades, months, or are just getting started, these lists should help you pursue Cannabis more effectively and with more enjoyment than just "figuring it out" on your own.

Cannabis Preparation Checklist:

1. Explore specific compound recommendations from actual Cannabis experts.
2. Determine which Cannabis compounds to consume.
3. Determine how much of each compound to consume.
4. Learn to prefer consumption methods that are "harm-reductive" in relation to smoking.
5. Buy products with enough compounds to provide for recommended dosages.
6. If you have concerns about psychoactive effects, be sure to consult Cannabis experts who can help strategize the exploration of compounds that are psychoactive. For example: a medical professional who is a Cannabis expert might know that a person who is new to Cannabis will be likely to experience pain until they

are able to tolerate enough psychoactive effects to consume larger doses of THC.

7. People who are new to Cannabis will likely need help strategizing ways they can explore increasing their personal tolerance. New people should start with small doses until they feel prepared to face the psychoactive effects of larger doses. If too large a dose is consumed, then they might consider reducing future dosages. People who feel like they "took too much" should also know that they will be just fine and that they should try their best to get some sleep or distract their thoughts until the effects are reduced. Cannabis is nonlethal in terms of any "Cannabis overdose."

8. Planning for initial dosings and personal tolerance is an important step in helping people learn to be as successful as possible in their pursuit of Cannabis. Without proper planning, someone may want to give up and seek "easier" or "more affordable" alternatives that could be more dangerous or less beneficial than Cannabis. Cannabis usage can be difficult for some people to learn, but it can and does save lives by avoiding other less beneficial alternatives.

9. Track and journal ongoing usage. Know how much dosages cost so that adjustments can be made if affordability or spending becomes too much of a financial burden. Determine appropriate dosage sizes for daytime and nighttime, the need or desire to take days off from dosing (Tolerance "T-breaks"), and which consumption methods might be best whether long-term or short-term consumption is expected. Short-term and long-term considerations are covered in Consideration 12.

Troubleshooting Tips

1. Start slow when exploring beginner tolerance levels to psychoactive effects.

2. If overwhelmed, reduce dosing levels until psychoactive effects become more tolerable. Many "tolerance issues" can be solved

immediately with good advice. Some people might require personal exploration (therapy) on how to overcome their specific "tolerance issues." This would be the case if a "tolerance issue" cannot be solved with quick Cannabis advice.

3. Nobody is required to consume Cannabis. If a Cannabis expert recommends Cannabis and someone is unable to "tolerate it," then this person will need to weigh their "Cannabis tolerance" against the effects and side effects that other alternatives will bring into their life. If someone hates Cannabis, then they are welcome to not consume it, pursue other treatments, or not consume anything at all. However, if it is recommended to someone by a medical professional who is a Cannabis expert, then it should be taken seriously in spite of anyone's personal preference or personal reasons as to why they don't like Cannabis. In the end, though, every person is responsible for their own suffering, and no one is required to choose Cannabis if they don't want to.

4. Be in a comfortable place while exploring tolerance levels. Learn to enjoy the navigation of personal tolerance levels. Recognize that personal tolerance levels can potentially fluctuate outside your comfort zone based on factors such as daily metabolism, method of consumption, and strain and/or regularity of dosings. Embrace that and discover which experiences you most prefer.

5. The effects of THC can seem more or less noticeable based on preexisting THC levels in the body. *Tolerance* is usually the word used to describe this, but in this book I have chosen to teach "tolerance" as something to **overcome**, not something to **maintain**.

The following two examples show that just because an experienced consumer is familiar with high doses, it's no guarantee that they won't experience the same tolerance issues of an inexperienced consumer. It also shows that tolerance issues might not be experienced at all by either type of person.

A first-time consumer consumes 1 gram/20%THC/Flower. This would be about 200mg/THC.

Outcome: This person may be at risk of feeling nauseous and/or become overwhelmed by psychoactive effects . . . or they might tolerate this amount just fine.

A longtime consumer of more than ten years who typically consumes 400mg/THC on most days, takes a two-week "tolerance break." This person might be very aware and comfortable with psychoactive effects, but their body might not so easily adjust. After their two-week break, they consume a joint that contains half the amount of THC they were used to consuming each day.

Outcome: This person may be at risk of feeling nauseous and/or becoming overwhelmed by psychoactive effects . . . or they might tolerate this amount just fine. Experienced consumers can still have tolerance issues that would be comparable to the experiences of inexperienced first-time consumers.

Consideration 12

Is It Safe to Smoke Flower and How Much Should You Plan to Smoke?

Occasional/Short-Term/Small-Dose Strategies for Smoking Cannabis

If you don't plan to regularly consume Cannabis, it probably doesn't matter a whole lot how you choose to occasionally consume it. If you only rarely consume flower, you should pursue products that have been tested for contaminants. If tested products are not available, then learn to inspect quality and potency as best you can. You should also study Cannabis compounds and the psychoactive effects of THC—preferably prior to consumption, but definitely if long-term use is expected or recommended.

Smoking flower should be mostly avoided whenever possible. Smoking flower is not recommended because there are better methods for consuming Cannabis compounds. Smoking small amounts may not cause any problems, but inhaling anything that isn't beneficial into the lungs should be avoided or reduced as much as possible. The main reason smoking isn't the best is because edible and concentrated products have many reasons for being better methods of consumption, as shown by the rankings found in Consideration 6. Is smoking really as damaging as some people might imagine, though? Probably not.

Smoking flower doesn't usually become problematic for people who only consume small or occasional dosages. Smoking is more time-consuming and smells and tastes like ash with only small hints of flavor from wasted terpenes. Smoking is far less flavorful than using vaporizer devices, consuming edibles, or vaporizing concentrated compounds. That said, we should be free to consume Cannabis compounds however we choose.

It doesn't matter how famous someone is or how long someone has been smoking countless joints every day. Smoking flower shouldn't be promoted because we should be promoting better methods of consumption. People should be allowed to promote smoking if they want, but anyone who promotes smoking should at least consider promoting other methods of consumption. Anyone who is actually interested in helping people improve their health or general well-being should aim to promote better products, better consumption methods, and better preferred resources for ongoing Cannabis education.

Being as "harm-reductive" as possible is always good. Most of us probably won't need to start taking frequent/high-dose/long-term considerations until reaching somewhere around 500+mg/ THC/Day. However, people with existing breathing issues may want to avoid inhalation completely (smoking or vaporizing) unless a medical professional who regularly prescribes Cannabis to people who experience similar conditions specifically recommends this.

Being "harm-reductive" by avoiding smoking is beneficial, even if it doesn't "technically matter" because someone only plans to pursue occasional, small, or short-term consumption of Cannabis. Harm reduction should be taught and shared by everyone who cares to provide better suggestions to the people around them. Nobody is required to live by what they teach, but anyone recommending or distributing Cannabis should either educate people themselves or recommend other educational resources if they are unable to provide expert-level advice.

Be aware that if your consumption levels start rising closer to that 2.5g/20%Flower/Day mark (500mg/THC), you may need to start taking a more long-term/high-dose approach to your Cannabis consumption.

Frequent/Long-Term/High-Dose Strategies for Smoking Cannabis

If someone is consuming upwards of 500+mg/THC/day, they should probably consider consuming Cannabis pretty much any other way besides smoking flower. People concerned with their health and well-being should not be inhaling smoke from burned material. Smoking is less bioavailable, tastes worse, and requires far more preparation and cleaning than vaporizing, edibles or concentrated compounds.

Once habits are formed, we tend to keep doing the same things until something becomes an actual problem. We should avoid getting stuck maintaining less beneficial habits just because something is enjoyable. We also shouldn't continue poor habits just because other people do it or if other personal habits in the past were more toxic. Examples of this are people who have a previous history with escaping other non beneficial substances or habits and decide that current consumptions or habits aren't worth changing because at least things are "better than they used to be." People should aim to form and reform the best habits they can in food, Cannabis, or anything else they consume.

Excessive consumption is sometimes recommended in very specific situations. If someone is recommended to consume 1,000+mg/THC/day, they would need to consume 6g/20%THCFlower. Inhaling six FULL GRAMS of burned material into the lungs is never advisable. People are simply far better off if they can reduce or replace the habit of smoking by leveraging other forms of consumption instead. Nobody is required to completely quit smoking—it is a personal choice to make—but everyone should aspire to minimize or eliminate smoking as much as possible. If someone is actually trying to help themselves, they should avoid inhaling burned smoke that could create problems.

On another note, smoking Cannabis can become extremely time-consuming. Smoking 6 grams of anything is extremely time-consuming. Preparing flower, rolling joints, cleaning glass pipes/bongs, and sitting down to smoke 6 grams is going to eat up some time. Other consumption methods taste better, save time, and make it way easier to consume daily recommendations without having to fight through heated smoke that can become problematic. It may be enjoyable for people to participate in smoking "rituals" such as preparation, cleaning, and smoking, but people who learn to improve their consumption will live with the benefits of better flavor, more time, and better bioavailability. If someone actually enjoys Cannabis, then why waste so many good aspects that Cannabis has to offer?

After learning to appreciate and prefer other consumption methods, smoking can really start to lose its appeal. Smoking joints is cleaner than smoking dirty pipes and bongs. At least the flavors and smells of joints aren't completely overtaken by overwhelming flavors of ash, nasty pipe resin, or dirty bong water. As for the lungs, people might enjoy getting some deep breathing they don't normally get (if someone is not active), but lungs definitely prefer oxygen-rich inhalation over smoke. Deep breathing is important, but it shouldn't require inhalation of any substance just to make sure it takes place every single day.

Pre-made edibles don't require entire smoke sessions. Vaporizers stay cleaner longer, and they vaporize rather than burn. Vaporizers are also much easier to clean compared to various pipes and bongs. Concentrate consumption requires far less total inhalation into the lungs compared to flower. Rolling joints, cleaning pipes, and cleaning bongs steal valuable time from people. And most of us would probably prefer better flavor, saving time, and reducing health risks.

No matter what you choose: "May your journey and decisions serve you well."

Conclusion

You finished my book! First of all, thank you. Every time we share Cannabis education with the world, we are one step closer to universal homegrowing for everyone. Now that you understand Cannabis, it should be much easier to notice how dangerous and destructive anti-Cannabis advice actually is. Homegrowing and consuming Cannabis is a natural human right that we all deserve. Homegrowing should be universally allowed for recreational, medical, spiritual, or religious purposes. Universal homegrowing laws should be recognized, established, and protected forever. No laws should be allowed to be more strict than universally protected homegrowing laws that should be developed and established to protect the freedom of us all.

Those who speak down to Cannabis consumers should be aware that forcing their opinions of Cannabis on others is disrespectful, ignorant of others, spiritually oppressive, and religiously oppressive, and it should be viewed as blatant discrimination that could lead to criminal charges. People who consume Cannabis deserve to have the same protection as anyone else. The world should have never allowed religious opinions to dictate the personal consumptions of individuals, whether they are religious or not. Opinions that do not support Cannabis literally perpetuate mass suffering. Humans deserve the freedom and protection to homegrow Cannabis without financial penalty and without religious dominance of the role or purpose of Cannabis in other people's life.

If it were up to me, homegrowing would be universally established, protected forever, and effective immediately. As for you personally? I wish you a safe lifetime in your own pursuit of Cannabis wherever you might be. Cannabis isn't legal everywhere just yet, and there are people who will decide to ruin someone else's life for choosing Cannabis. Be aware of your environment and recognize that dead-end debates do exist. Religious debates are not worth pursuing and should only be met by sharing educational resources. I do not recommend debating with people who actively try not to be convinced of Cannabis. If someone isn't trying to understand the reality of Cannabis through education, then it's not worth debating with them. People who still try to debate the benefits of Cannabis today often have no intention of "losing their perspective," and their main objective may be to ignore every good point you could possibly give. If someone isn't willing to do their own research, don't waste your time. Live your life however you choose, and if people don't like it, you get to decide whether to share Cannabis education with them or separate yourself completely from individuals who choose to perpetuate disrespectful remarks against Cannabis.

To wrap things up, I wish you the best of luck in your pursuit of Cannabis. If you already consume Cannabis, I hope this book helps you continue that pursuit to the best of your ability. If you don't already consume Cannabis, keep in mind that it may be helpful in your future to pursue the consumption of Cannabis compounds sooner rather than later. Whatever your case might be, stay safe, be happy, and help spread the word that the benefits of Cannabis are for everyone.

Appendix

How Cannabis Started, How It's Going, and What Should Come Next

How Cannabis Started

Cannabis-related plants have been evolving on Earth for millions of years. After humans discovered Cannabis thousands of years ago, they have been consuming Cannabis ever since. Cannabis has been consumed for medical benefits, religious practices and personal preference. Humans didn't create Cannabis, but we have been studying it for thousands of years. Cannabis has always been beneficial, and today it's more beneficial than ever.

The demonization of Cannabis didn't become an issue until Roman Christians decided it was God's "Master Plan" to convert, dominate, or destroy every non-Christian religion in the world. Christians have been the most destructive force to Cannabis in the history of the world. Christians tend to view other Christians as good people, which they certainly can be, but the truth is that the core of Christian agendas were literally designed and continue to actively convert or destroy anything or anyone who doesn't obey laws that are maintained by their modern-day prophets, popes, and other religious leaders. The pursuits of Christian religions today are no different than the ancient Romans' pursuit of literal world domination. Christians are known to view other non-Christian cultures and people as less intelligent and dangerous for any pursuit of Cannabis. Any non-Christian religions that also prohibit Cannabis are also guilty of manipulation, corruption, and contributing to the historical mass suffering of everyone.

How It's Going

Today, the benefits of Cannabis are known to be beneficial to everyone. Cannabis is still illegal in many places, but religious dominance is now recognized as oppressive, undesirable, and destructive when it prevents individuals from understanding that the benefits of Cannabis do exist and that these benefits are meant for everyone. The difference today is that we now know that people without legal access to Cannabis experience more suffering than people who are able to pursue the benefits of Cannabis. It's only a matter of time before we regain our personal freedom to pursue the benefits of Cannabis.

What Should Come Next

What should legalization look like? Should Cannabis be allowed recreationally, medically, spiritually, or religiously? The correct answer is "all of the above." Everyone should have the right and protected freedom to pursue Cannabis. Everyone should be allowed to homegrow Cannabis, and testing should be made available to anyone who wishes to sell their products. Homegrowing should become the global standard for human rights to personal freedom in their pursuit of Cannabis.

About the Author

D avid Putvin was born February 29, 1992, and he was raised in Copperton, Utah, USA. Cannabis became important to him once he realized that Cannabis prohibition significantly increases the mass suffering of everyone on the planet. David's passion in life is to help create sustainable building projects that improve general wellness, promote self-mastery, and provide freedom in the exploration of psychoactive experiences. His hope is that the success of these sustainable building projects will lead to increased acceptance and understanding of the significance of psychoactive freedom for everyone, no matter who tries to dominate the reality of human existence that we all share.

CPSIA information can be obtained
at www.ICGtesting.com
Printed in the USA
BVHW050539100323
660081BV00013B/1239